Loss and Grief

Loss and Grief

Personal Stories of Doctors and Other Healthcare Professionals

Edited by
MATTHEW LOSCALZO AND
MARSHALL FORSTEIN

Co-edited by
LINDA A. KLEIN

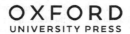
OXFORD
UNIVERSITY PRESS

OXFORD
UNIVERSITY PRESS

Oxford University Press is a department of the University of Oxford. It furthers
the University's objective of excellence in research, scholarship, and education
by publishing worldwide. Oxford is a registered trade mark of Oxford University
Press in the UK and certain other countries.

Published in the United States of America by Oxford University Press
198 Madison Avenue, New York, NY 10016, United States of America.

Library of Congress Cataloging-in-Publication Data
Names: Loscalzo, Matthew, editor. | Forstein, Marshall, 1949– editor. | Klein, Linda A., co-editor.
Title: Loss and grief : personal stories of doctors and other healthcare professionals /
edited by Matthew Loscalzo and Marshall Forstein ; co-edited by Linda A. Klein.
Other titles: Loss and grief (Loscalzo)
Description: New York, NY : Oxford University Press, [2023] |
Includes bibliographical references and index.
Identifiers: LCCN 2022010880 (print) | LCCN 2022010881 (ebook) |
ISBN 9780197524534 (paperback) | ISBN 9780197524558 (epub) | ISBN 9780197524565 (other)
Subjects: MESH: Grief | Physicians—psychology | Health
Personnel—psychology | Adaptation, Psychological | Personal Narrative
Classification: LCC BF575.G7 L676 2023 (print) | LCC BF575.G7 (ebook) |
NLM BF 575.G7 | DDC 155.937—dc23/eng/20220608
LC record available at https://lccn.loc.gov/2022010880
LC ebook record available at https://lccn.loc.gov/2022010881

DOI: 10.1093/med/9780197524534.001.0001

1 3 5 7 9 8 6 4 2

Printed by Marquis, Canada

Thank you Joanne Mortimer, Concetta Greco Loscalzo, and family, for your love and inspiration.

Thank you Marshall Forstein and Linda A. Klein, for your creativity, fearlessness, and patience.

Thank you Susan Dale Block, for your generosity of spirit and exploration of uncharted territory.

Thank you to all the courageous and compassionate people who have the audacity to demand that people be treated with empathy, dignity, and respect, including those who may not have earned it yet. These losses we can control.
—Matthew Loscalzo, LCSW

To all of my patients who have taught me how to bear suffering with grace and wisdom; my parents who made life possible, joyful, passionate, and full of hope; my children who taught me how to love unconditionally and supported me through difficult times; and my husband, now gone, who made me a better, more loving person than I had ever imagined possible.
—Marshall Forstein, MD

To my Dad Hal, for teaching me the difference.
To Michael and Michelle, for teaching me fun is the best thing to have.
To Chip, Eila, Skye, and Charlie: you are the best things I've ever done. I love you a trillion billion.
And to my Mom Esther, the light that shines on me: you are and always will be my hero.
—Linda A. Klein, JD

Contents

Acknowledgments

To the courageous authors, all of whom chose duty over escape.

It is not possible to adequately thank colleagues, friends, and family for their feedback, guidance, and support. Everyone listed below made a positive impact on the book and for that we are forever grateful.

We also acknowledge Lynn and Howard Behar, Sheri and Les Biller, Courtney Bitz, Emily Black, George A. Bonanno, Barry Bultz, Karen Clark, William Dale, Bonnie DuPont, Linda L. Emanuel, Lawrence (Khari) Farrell, Mike Feddersen, Carrie Fogliani-Richards, Scott David Farrell-Forstein, Susan Golant, Emma Hodgdon (Oxford University Press), Chip James, Audrey Kapuscinski, Michelle L. Klein, Andrea Knobloch (Oxford University Press), Juee Kotwal, Erik Kronstadt, Alexandra and Victor Levine, Andrea Lynch, Henry Mager, Lori McGee, Annette Mercurio, Mary-Frances O'Connor, Holly Prigerson, Claudia Robertson, Don Rosenstein, Daniela Salinas, Natalie Schnaitmann, Fabian Shalini, the Simone family, Philip Vassallo, James Waisman, and Joanne Weingarten.

About the Editors

Matthew Loscalzo, LCSW, APOS Fellow, is a founding Executive Director and Emeritus Professor of Supportive Care Medicine and Professor of Population Sciences at City of Hope. Professor Loscalzo was President of the American Psychosocial Oncology Society and the Association of Oncology Social Workers, and he has held leadership positions at Memorial Sloan-Kettering Cancer Center, Johns Hopkins Oncology Center, Eastern Virginia Medical School, and the Rebecca and John Moores Cancer Center at the University of California, San Diego. He has been a consultant to multiple major cancer organizations on how to build supportive care programs, implement new processes, and enhance staff engagement through his unique staff leadership model. His clinical interests and scholarly contributions are gender-based medicine, strengths-based approaches to psychotherapies, pain management, problem-based distress screening, and the creation of supportive care programs.

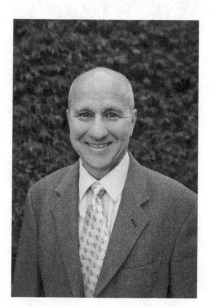

Marshall Forstein, MD, is a psychiatrist with more than 40 years of experience. He is the co-founder of one of the first HIV Collaborative Care Clinics at the Cambridge Health Alliance (CHA), a public-sector Harvard-affiliated teaching hospital. Dr. Forstein has been Medical Director of Mental Health at the Fenway Health Center, one of the largest health centers dedicated to the LGBTQ communities. For nineteen years, he was the training director of the Psychiatry Residency Program at CHA, where he also served as Acting Chair of the Department of Psychiatry and Vice Chair for Education and Training. He has been active on governmental and professional organization committees and task forces in the areas of HIV/AIDS and gender and sexuality, and he has written and taught nationally. He is currently on the teaching faculty at CHA/Harvard Medical School and maintains a private practice.

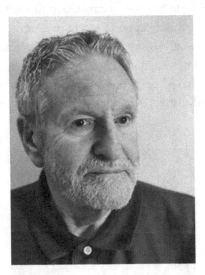

Linda A. Klein, JD, began her professional career as an attorney. Out of law school, she was selected to do a coveted federal clerkship for the Honorable Florence-Marie Cooper, District Court, and went on to work with Fortune 500 companies at a prestigious global law firm. At age 25, Ms. Klein, her father, and three siblings watched their 55-year-old mom die from breast cancer. They received no guidance around end-of-life care or what was to come after, never mind language they could use to help each other heal. As a result, she changed careers. Ms. Klein was recruited by the Department of Supportive Care Medicine, City of Hope to oversee the Sheri & Les Biller Patient and Family Resource Center, where she developed a large number of integrated interdisciplinary programs focused on enhancing strengths and resiliency in cancer patients and their families. She also contributed significantly to the *Science of Caring* portion of Medical Grand Rounds and assumed a leadership role in building the institution-wide advance care planning initiative. She currently leads bereavement support groups at Our House, one of the largest nonprofit grief centers in California.

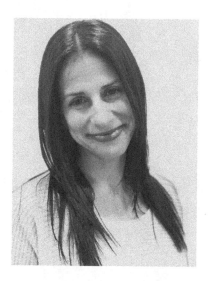

Contributors

Craig D. Blinderman, MD

Susan D. Block, MD

Marshall Forstein, MD

Mitch Golant, PhD

John Halporn, MD

Wendy S. Harpham, MD, FACP

Linda A. Klein, JD

Cheryl Krauter, MFT

Matthew Loscalzo, LCSW, APOS Fellow

Damon Madison, EMBA

Joan Heller Miller, EdM

Ken Miller, MD

Steven T. Rosen, MD, FACP, FASCO

Julia H. Rowland, PhD

Lidia Schapira, MD

Amy N. Ship, MD, MA, FACP

Joseph V. Simone, MD (1935–2021)

Patricia Ann Sheahan Simone, RN, BA

Cy A. Stein, MD, PhD

Fredda Wasserman, MA, MPH, LMFT

Introduction

Marshall Forstein

This collection of personal narratives is just that: stories intended to chronicle the journeys of a small number of health clinicians and other professionals who have been struck by personal illness and/or loss. During the development of each person's story, the editors and some of the authors who were themselves contributing to the collective reflections met almost monthly for more than a year to coach, support, critique, and love each other as we wrote and experienced the pain of telling and retelling our individual stories. What these stories do not assume is that there are answers to the universal experiences of loss and grief, courage, and survival implicit in the telling. While the past is gone, the meaning of it, however, is forever in flux, forever being worked and reworked in our conscious and unconscious minds. Each memory is a redoing of what it represents and brings forth within our sense of ourselves and in our relationships with one another. Grief challenges us physically, emotionally, and psychologically to recast the loss again and again, sometimes for the rest of our remaining consciousness. And, in recasting the past and the passage of time, refashioning memory to meet the needs of the moment in which the lost object and our response to it either helps us to move forward in our life or keeps us stuck, unable to engage with a future that requires acceptance of giving up the life lived before.

For the editors as well, the resonance of each story with our own has been both a burden and gift, an inescapable reflection of the connectedness we all share as human beings.

We asked contributors to distinguish loss from grief. Loss is what happened, forever immutable. Even if what has been lost is somehow, in some way, recovered, such as a body part or function, we are never the same. Loss of a loved, treasured person, even one with whom there remains some ambivalence, creates a void that can never be truly filled. Loss is that which is gone forever as it was. Grief is what we do with the loss: how and where we feel it and how we try, sometimes more successfully than others, to move through that loss to regain some footing in our life remaining. We cannot choose to forget what is most painful, nor might we want to, and, with time and age, we cannot sometimes choose to remember those aspects of what we have lost that recede into time itself. What comes through in each story is the recognition that in our grief, and in memories, we keep present in our minds and hearts that which we have lost.

We are reminded by these recollections that illness, death, loss, and grief are different for each of us, and we experience them according to who we are and what we have gone through. Illness takes many turns, and death comes to some expectedly or not, sudden, or prolonged. We cannot look to our bookshelves for the definitive experience. If the universe or a higher power has indeed a master plan and way to be in the world or is watching as those we love leave it, it is yet to be revealed. As we wait, having those we love around us to bear witness, to listen, to hold us and be still with us is perhaps the most of what we can hope.

The time elapsed from the onset of the loss/or illness to the start of writing about it varied greatly, but for none did the process of grieving and making meaning finish, even in some cases with a significant passage of time. While there was an eagerness to finish the account because it was painful, there was also a reluctance to say the story was finished for it is not, even when we finally let that story go to the editors to meet publishing deadlines.

One might say that the brain has a linear cognitive framework of time and memory, but the human heart and mind know no such boundaries. How is it that a few bars of music, a photograph, or a line from a poem—often that might have had nothing to do with the actual experience—can elicit a cascade of emotion, even years later, one so powerful as to stop us in place and make time disappear? How do we learn to welcome and treasure both the tears and sadness, memories of love and intricate, complex relationships? How do we separate the story from the storyteller, the art from the artist, or, as Yeats said, "How can we know the dancer from the dance?"[1]

Naïvely, perhaps, the individual writing and collective process was more complicated and difficult than expected: while the suffering we minister to as physicians, nurses, psychologists, and social workers is the daily fare, writing about the exposure and vulnerability of one's personal suffering after having been "educated" in a specialty that expects you to deal with that on one's own revealed insights into some of the very failures of how we educate and train healthcare professionals. The COVID pandemic further highlighted the internalization of expectations. Dr. Rieux says in Camus's portentous novel *The Plague*,[2] "The thing was to do your job as it should be done." Drilled into us in training is the "prime directive," the ethical responsibility of patient care and that one should deal with personal things on one's one time. What time? At what cost? How?

We know that professionals are reluctant to seek support and, even more commonly, mental health treatment when the personal suffering impairs even that prime directive. While the stories are greatly variable, each of them resonates with feelings of loss, grief, shame, guilt, fear of being seen as incompetent to "handle it all," and sometimes despair, anxiety, and emotional paralysis. The group struggled with how to give honest and sometimes difficult feedback for fear of contributing to the experiences that were in all cases challenging at best and, at worst, despairing. Each of us was asked to let others hear and see us in a very vulnerable and often re-traumatizing way. It was as though each of us opened our personal Pandora's box, unleashing deep, visceral emotions of pain and suffering while trying to regain some footing, some hope that the next day, the next week, and the future would be easier. For some, at various moments, feeling tentative and being open led to an increased sense of vulnerability with its perceived risks to profession and relationships. For others, this increased sense of authenticity became armor against the possibility of risks in the professional and personal realms. Ironically, fears of weakness led to feelings of greater invulnerability; secrets and shame gave way to unexpected inspiration and empathic connection. What does it mean that what might be perceived and feared as weakness may lead to unanticipated strength? As editors, we struggled to tread lightly but firmly to make suggestions about the writing itself, to push gently to deepen the disclosure of feelings open or defended. As authors as well as editors, we understood what was being asked, and the those who answered the call to contribute gave of their most personal selves, for which we are so very grateful.

Readers, especially other healthcare professionals, might wonder why we agreed to do this. It is not clear that any of us have coherent answers. For some, the process was not completed. The process of writing itself leads to a new perspective, sometimes helpful and sometimes not. It might be fair to say that more writing has been done about the human experience of love and loss than is ever published. The act of writing itself helps to access parts of the mind that remain in the shadows of memory, both visceral and cognitive. It is both selfish and selfless. Even those stories that are seen by others are worked and reworked both for the art and for the overcoming of the fears of putting out into the world what can then never be recalled. Like any artist or poet, once public, the author no longer controls the meanings that their heart's work intended. We may agree that a color is called green, but how do we really know (or is it even possible?) what the other sees is the same?

The stories written in this collection were a draft, one of the many, perhaps unending (or upending) versions telling of the experience. Some stories were written in one setting, others over many weeks or months as the writer lost and regained footing along the tale's trail. The shame, the sadness and weeping, the anger and guilt, and the shame of feeling relief of the pain and suffering for ourselves or those we love(d) and the "weakness" of not being able to manage it all echo through these stories. The reflection seen when looking in the emotional mirror is not about seeing oneself, but seeing many parts and versions of the self, as though one is standing in front of a mirror with a mirror behind reflecting an infinite number of selves back and forth, not only in consciousness but also in dreams. The contributors of this collection have been forever changed by the experiences written here and by the process of writing and sharing those experiences as well. The editors, too, as contributors of our own stories, have been forever changed by the privilege of sharing the process of sitting with the pain and angst of bringing the narrative to this manuscript. We have witnessed incredible courage—and felt some of our own— as we asked nothing more of the contributors than we did of ourselves. We know that these stories are now in your hands and, hopefully, in your hearts.

Some readers might resonate with their own painful experiences and memories, and others might wonder how they might, and perhaps will, imagine their own future when this inevitable aspect of being human—loss and grief—strikes them, too.

References

1 Yeats, W. B. "Among School Children." Published in a collection of his poems *The Tower*, in 1928.
2 Camus, A. *The Plague*, published in French in 1947 and English in 1948.

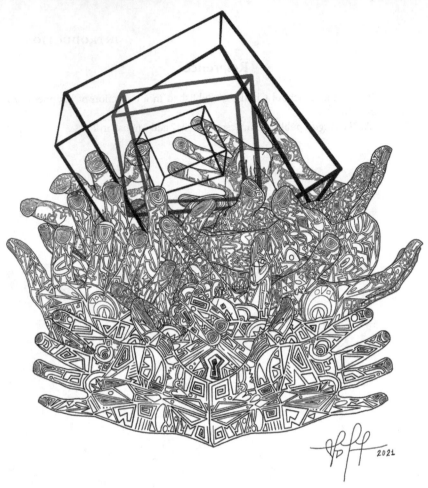

"Pandora's Unboxing." Humans, regardless of varying myths from many cultures, have been plagued by illness, loss, and grief since the beginning of time. In Greek mythology, in one version of the story, all manner of evil and misery were contained in a jar and released into the world unwittingly by Pandora, who opened the jar (later a box, as described Erasmus in the sixteenth century). In later versions, the box contained not evils but blessings, which would have been preserved for humanity had Pandora's curiosity not let them out. But Hope, which lingered at the edge of the box, was shut in before she could escape, providing solace henceforth to those in pain and suffering. This illustration allows us to meditate, as do the very personal narratives in this compendium, on hope in a world full of inevitable loss and grief. The deeply personal stories that follow represents courageous and compassionate insights into many of our most atavistic fears but also our greatest hopes.

Source: Scott David Farrell-Forstein, "Pandora's Unboxing." The graphic of "Pandora's Unboxing," is an original print created by Scott Farrell-Forstein, the son of Marshall Forstein, one of the editors of and contributors to this volume. In managing his own grief after the death of one of his fathers to cancer, he was soon faced with a cancer diagnosis for his other father as well. Together, he and his dad supported each other through their shared grief and his father's successful cancer treatment. He also chose to contribute to the book by providing the painting featured on the front cover of this volume. Scott is a full-time artist working in multimedia pen and ink, paint, construction, and music composition and production.

1

An Oncologist Reflects on Loss and the Culture of Medicine

Lidia Schapira

As a patient I would want a doctor who cares for me as a person, wouldn't you?

If I were diagnosed with a serious, life-altering illness I would want a doctor whose presence gave me comfort. I would endow them with the power to lift my spirits when they called or walked into my room. Of course, I would also want them to have scientific expertise and technical skills, but I would most cherish their ability to attend to my existential and emotional needs. My doctor would analyze my data *and* listen to me, even bargain with me when tough decisions need to be made. I would want to be in the hands of somebody who kept me feeling safe from the chaos, indignity, and suffering that accompanies disease.

I chose a career in medical oncology in large measure because I wanted to be *that* person for my future patients. I didn't think about the emotional labor it would take to cultivate and sustain such a therapeutic presence or consider the toll of cumulative losses and constant exposure to the suffering of others. It was not addressed during medical training, and attending physicians never talked about their lived experience of loss or shared how they dealt with professional losses. I seriously underestimated the effort and training that was required in addition to vocation and determination.

As students and trainees during residency and fellowship, my peers and I simply packed up our bundled emotions at the end of a shift or rotation and dumped them somewhere or shelved them someplace within our psyche with other traumas, to be dealt with later. As I write these words, I have flashbacks to moments of unresolved loss, such as when a beloved internist who served as a clinical role model during medical school died by suicide and there was silence. Or when a fellow resident took a leave of absence due to severe depression and we avoided talking about it directly, instead commiserating about the lack of light and the bitter cold of a Boston winter. My peers and I were encouraged to cultivate detachment and lighten the load through exercise, the pursuit of hobbies, and time spent with family and friends.

I was a medical resident in the early 1980s, at the height of the AIDS epidemic. We were immersed in a demoralized, distressed, and overworked professional workforce, where therapeutic failure was the norm. The organizational culture was not sufficiently nimble or dynamic to recognize the toll this epidemic was taking on the mental health of nurses, respiratory therapists, physicians, and trainees who spent their waking hours surrounded by suffering and loss. The concept of burnout was known at the time—in fact, Dr. Virginia Maslach published her inventory and survey tools in 1981[1]—and yet academic physicians were slow to recognize the symptoms of this syndrome within their ranks and slow to implement supportive interventions to mitigate stress and emotional exhaustion. Medical training reinforced my instinct to keep my experiences to myself, and, although I welcomed the superficial camaraderie of peers and supervisors, I did not look for opportunities to process my emotions or reflect on my experience of loss and suffering.

After residency I took a gap year and worked 9–5 at a community hospital, traveled, jogged, and skied before starting an oncology fellowship. Cancer medicine combined the intellectual excitement of scientific discovery with the profoundly humanitarian work of helping people who were fighting to stay alive. New therapeutics offered possibilities for cure and longevity where none had been previously imagined. Training was intense, but the intellectual and human rewards made it manageable, indeed exhilarating.

I learned from extraordinary clinicians who were supportive of trainees and not only brilliant but also caring and compassionate. A senior attending instructed me on the first day of my inpatient rotation to make sure that I visited dying hospitalized patients at least twice a day. He told me it was important to convey my respect and caring to the patient's family and warned me not to forget to do a careful physical examination and do my best every day to maintain comfort. My research mentor was a star in his field and the kindest physician imaginable. He was loved by patients with sickle cell disease, a terrible condition that leads to painful crises and for which there was at the time no effective treatment or cure. It was clear that his compassion for the suffering of his patients provided the inspiration for his research and that he had earned the trust and loyalty of entire families. His kindness extended to the most junior members of his team, as I learned when he offered to babysit for my infant daughter so I could attend a lab meeting.

Our division was blessed with two amazing social workers who looked after our patients—and us, too. I remember walking the long hallways of the Brigham and Women's Hospital with Martha, just telling her what was on my mind, organically and unprompted, and always feeling better afterward. She helped me prepare for a weekend conversation with the five-year-old daughter of my leukemic patient who couldn't walk because chemotherapy had destroyed her sense of balance. She helped me understand how a patient experiences the trauma of watching their roommate die in hospital. She even listened as I told her about a new relationship and humored me as I listed a bunch of concerns.

When I finished my fellowship training, the demoralization and emotional exhaustion among US oncologists had reached an intolerable level. This was captured in a survey conducted by the Editor-in-Chief and published in the *Journal of Clinical Oncology*. This informal poll showed that more than half of responding oncologists were burned out. The cumulative and unresolved grief associated with repeated losses threatened to destroy the workforce.[2] The profession was duly warned.

At that point in my medical career, I had experienced a significant number of patient deaths. I'm wondering if it was in the dozens or hundreds? The answer probably depends on how we count them: just witnessed, or we were involved in the care of the person who died? How involved, and for how long? Had we ever had a meaningful conversation, or was I the intern-on-call who responded to an unsuccessful code? Loss was routinized, and it took years for me to realize that losses occurred at multiple levels and required acknowledgment and time for recovery.

Loss Gets Personal

But it was not until I was a second-year fellow in hematology-oncology that I experienced the gut-wrenching punch of personal loss. My father was diagnosed with an advanced and incurable brain tumor. An accomplished physician-scientist beloved by his patients and students, his symptoms had been misdiagnosed for more than a year. His doctors didn't want to use the word cancer, and I felt they abandoned him at a critical moment of need. My father and I had always found a way to handle difficult topics, even if it meant reaching an agreement to avoid a certain conversation because it caused anxiety or because we could not reconcile our points of view. I remember that his mood and mental status fluctuated and were not at baseline as a result of his tumor, and I wondered if that contributed to the collusion among family and professionals who withheld the diagnosis and prognostic information.

He was my soul mate, but he was also 5,000 miles away. I traveled home as soon as I heard about the medical difficulties; seized the first moment when I thought he was oriented, alert, and capable of handling the news; and I told him. I blurted it out. You have a cancer in your brain that explains all the symptoms you've experienced in the past year. It is not curable. I showed your scans to the best neuroradiologists in the world and discussed the case with the most capable neurosurgeon, and there is nothing they can do. We can give you radiation and steroids, that may buy you a little time, but there is no guarantee that it will help. Perhaps you want to try it? He nodded his understanding and did not look surprised. I think we were both relieved to have broken through the toxic cloud of euphemisms and petty lies and excuses that had been previously rendered. I remember feeling calm and experiencing a sense of peace mixed with the early sting of anticipatory grief. We could not stop this process, but we would comfort each other until he took his last breath. And we did.

My father had a few weeks of radiation and steroids that only boosted his appetite and made him irritable, and this was not easy for my mother to handle alone. I returned for his final week and sat with him during his final hours. My father's passing left a deep hole at the core of my being that never healed and gave me a front row seat to the complex emotional choreography of mourning and grieving a major loss.

Secular philosophers write about the finitude of death, poets describe the inner landscape of loss and absence, psychologists explain the origins of sadness, and friends place their hands on your shoulder to comfort you when you cry. I don't remember asking for help or feeling I needed help. I thought the hurt would diminish with time and quickly returned to work without missing a beat. That was how we did it, that was how I did it.

Over the next several years, the culture of medicine evolved and so did the subculture of oncology. With more women in the field and advances in the science of psycho-oncology and palliative medicine, oncologists started talking about the human cost of intense exposure to suffering and therapeutic failure. Burnout mitigation strategies involved wellness practices and the integration of communication skills training. Informed by evidence, skills-based training was practical and empowering and included exercises designed to raise self-awareness and promote self-care. Participants informally shared stories of personal loss, and, in so doing, they assigned "meaning" to emotional experiences. Storytelling emerged as another antidote to burnout by allowing the narrator to process complex experiences that provided a physiologic outlet for stored emotions. In turn, readers had access to the lived experience of a colleague, and the narratives published in high-impact medical journals served to create a community that was more tolerant and mature.

I was an early enthusiast and champion of workshops and didactic exercises focused on the human side of cancer. As an attending physician, I made time during teaching rounds to discuss the experience of illness as well as the pathophysiology of disease. I invited patients to co-teach, used film clips to trigger discussion about communication, and I once read Margaret Edson's play "Wit" with a team of medical residents and students over a period of several weeks.[3] At my hospital I was known as the oncologist who taught others how to break bad news or how to have a difficult conversation with a dying patient. The relationships I crafted with patients were likely influenced by my deep connection to my father and our family's experience of illness and loss, although I honestly think I learned the most from patients and families under my care.

And, slowly, my professional losses mounted. At times I found it difficult to bear the responsibility of the role, knowing people trusted their lives to me. I fantasized about other lines of work ranging from a high-end travel agent to a college philosophy professor, especially at times when I wondered if my professional life was affecting my ability to be available and present for my family. There was a period when I felt my grief crested after three deaths, as if I had the capacity to store the full impact and then let it all out after a cycle was completed. When I first recognized this pattern, I was surprised and, years later, have no explanation. I took notice and prepared myself for that third one, and over time I allowed myself to experience the full gamut of feelings without labeling or censoring them, to let tears flow in a darkened movie theater before the start of the featured film, and to take time alone, preferably outdoors, to recalibrate when emotionally spent. I immersed myself in the literature of palliative medicine, mindful practice, and techniques that specifically addressed the role of emotion in the practice of medicine. With support from friends and a healthy dose of therapy, I gradually developed a more nuanced and mature capacity to absorb the emotional impact of my work.

Essays published in medical journals assured me that I was not alone. Physicians wrote about their losses, often describing their coming to terms with grief as a profoundly solitary experience. I was struck by descriptions of doctors sobbing in the shower or struggling to tell the kids what mommy does every day.[4] In time I learned to pivot professionally to reduce my clinical load and diversify my work portfolio and spend more time in research, teaching, and editing, all of which proved to be both meaningful and intellectually stimulating.

I started this chapter by asking the reader to reflect on the qualities and attributes they would seek or demand in their physician if they were diagnosed with a life-threatening illness. In posing the question, I was influenced by Anatole Broyard's exquisite illness memoir, "Intoxicated by My Illness." The author was a literary critic and used his witty and sharp writing style to critique the communication and professional demeanor of the oncologist who treated him for prostate cancer. In "The Patient Examines the Doctor," Broyard playfully laments the fact that his urologist did not see him as a person, that medical personnel coldly intervened in his life without appreciating him as a human being. He writes, "I'd like my doctor to scan *me*, to grope for my spirit as well as my prostate."[5]

I read Broyard's memoir in the mid '90s and wondered what it would have been like to be his treating physician. I frequently cited his work, and it inspired a collaboration with a patient that led to a short documentary exploring the patient–doctor relationship in the context of advanced illness. And in my quest to learn more about his experience, I called his widow and asked if we could meet to reflect on their lived experience. Over a lovely outdoor lunch in Cambridge, Massachusetts, Sandy Broyard spoke about her grief and answered my questions. In turn she wanted to know why I cared so much about the experience of patients and families and what sparked my curiosity. She summarized it beautifully as a philosopher's method for peeking into the vulnerability of human beings. The clinic was my lab, and the existential question of human suffering was the driver of my intellectual and personal pursuits.

Broyard's wish to have a doctor who knew *him* remains timeless and universal and was recently echoed in a moving essay published by a resident physician with metastatic osteosarcoma. Brooke Gabster, a beloved young physician at Stanford, wrote "I want my physicians to grow personally invested in my journey . . . now that I live and sleep with this cancer,

I selfishly want my team to do the same. I'm terrified my oncologists have grown immune to tragedy."[6] Even in our siloed and fragmented medical system, the connection between patient and doctor remains a central theme in stories of illness. The trusted doctor is invited to co-edit the patient's story of illness and, in so doing, finds meaning and purpose in their work.

There is no question that the labor inherent in crafting a therapeutic relationship is undervalued and that burnout in oncology is at an all-time high. A recent survey found nearly three-quarters of cancer clinicians in Ontario, Canada, met standardized criteria for burnout.[7] Interestingly, those surveyed identified organizational factors, such as having little control over schedule and practice, as drivers of burnout rather than the emotional toll of the work, as had been noted by the group surveyed decades earlier. However, if doctors are emotionally exhausted and frustrated it is hard to imagine they will take the time to sit and listen, to know the person with the disease, or even to recognize the need to mourn their losses. Ironically, the culture of medicine has evolved and is now more tolerant and open as medical educators have broadened the curriculum to include humanities and medical trainees have access to mental health services.

Physicians who became central figures in treating HIV/AIDS were recently invited to share their reflections in order to commemorate the forty-year anniversary of the epidemic.[8] Some spoke of "how dark it was," others used military metaphors referring to clinical work as being in "the trenches," or expressed outrage at societal taboos and indifference to the suffering of patients. And some spoke of being inspired and finding meaning in their work. It is too early to know how the COVID-19 pandemic has influenced a new generation of physicians, but there is no doubt that it has, and we will learn about the lasting effects in years to come.

Returning to the initial question of what I want and need in my physician if confronted with a life-threatening illness? I would want to know there is a human being inside the white coat. I would need somebody who appreciates language. I wouldn't ask for a great emotional investment in my case, as I understand that is a finite and valuable resource. But I would make sure there is a social worker or psychologist on the team with whom I could openly share my vulnerabilities and fears and who is willing to connect with me, human to human.

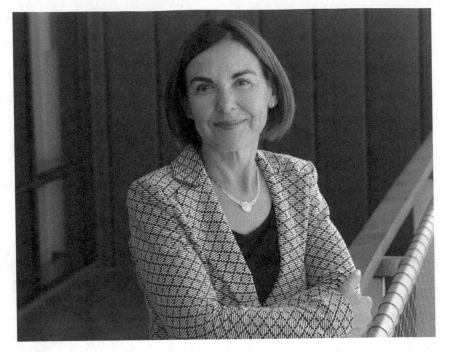

Author, 2018.

About the Author

Lidia Schapira, MD, is Professor of Medicine at Stanford and a medical oncologist with more than thirty years of experience. Originally from Argentina, Dr. Schapira trained in hematology and oncology at the Brigham and Women's Hospital in Boston. Her clinical practice is devoted to caring for women with breast cancer. She was a member of the Massachusetts General Hospital Breast Oncology Group from 2002 to 2016, and she served on the faculty at Harvard Medical School. Her research and scholarly interests address issues related to health equity in cancer care, psychosocial dimensions of cancer care, and meeting the needs of cancer survivors. At Stanford, Dr. Schapira serves as Director of the Cancer Survivorship Program and Associate Chief of the Office of Health Equity and Community Engagement. She served as Editor-in-Chief for Cancer.Net, the American Society of Clinical Oncology's website for the public, and is the current editor for the Art of Oncology section for the *Journal of Clinical Oncology*. She is the editor of *Essential of Cancer Survivorship: A Guide for Medical Professionals*.

References

1 Maslach C, Jackson SE. The measurement of experienced burnout. *J Organizational Behav*. 1981;2(2):99–113.
2 Whippen DA, Canellos GP. Burnout syndrome in the practice of oncology: Results of a random survey of 1,000 oncologists. *J Clin Oncol*. 1991 Oct;9(10):1916–1920.
3 Edson M. *Wit*. New York: Farar, Straus and Giroux; 1993.
4 Mark M. What mommy does. *J Clin Oncol*. 2017 Mar 10;35(8):912–913.
5 Broyard A. *Intoxicated By My Illness*. New York: Ballantine; 1992.
6 Gabster B. Resident report. *JAMA*. 2019 Nov 5;322(17):1653–1654.
7 Singh S, Farrelly A, Chan C, et al. Prevalence and workplace drivers of burnout in cancer care physicians in Ontario, Canada. *J Oncol Pract*. 2022 Jan;18(1):e60–e71.
8 Bayer R, Oppenheimer GM, Parisi V. Marking the 40th anniversary of the AIDS epidemic: American physicians look back. *N Engl J Med*. 2021 Sep 30;385(14):1251–1253.

2

On "Doing" Loss

Wendy S. Harpham

Growing up, I was not very good at "doing" loss. Consequently, as a young physician in my solo practice of internal medicine, I marveled at patients who seemed to thrive despite tragic diagnoses or life events while others seemed stuck in bitterness, anger, or grief. Knowing my white coat did not protect me in some magical way, I wondered how I'd respond. A question rattled around the back of my mind, unspoken: "How did you do it?"

Seven years after opening my practice, a cancer diagnosis yanked me to the other side of the stethoscope. I never asked, "Why me?" but wished I could turn back the clock to ask my patients about coping with adversity. Throughout those early years of my survivorship, I depended on my doctors and nurses, counseling, trial-and-error, spiritual faith, and cancer support groups to help me navigate a life that looked nothing like the one I'd planned for. In retrospect, had I known from the start the lessons learned over the years, I'd have spared myself a lot of unnecessary struggles.

I wish my illness hadn't dominated so much of my life. That said, I'm thankful for how the heightened uncertainty about my future shaped my priorities and parenting. As a physician, I've prized the lessons about healing, especially what loss taught me about living well. Here, I share a few stories about how I learned to tap into the power of grief and hope to find happiness after cancer rocked my universe[1] and how those lessons are now helping me through age-related losses and a recent diagnosis of aplastic anemia. May they serve your efforts to provide compassionate care to patients—and your efforts to respond in healthy ways to loss in your own life.

---

[1] Harpham, W. S. (2005). *Happiness in a storm*. New York: W.W. Norton.

My Story

From the moment I felt the call of medicine as a teenager, I envisioned fulfilling my passion through primary care. An irrepressible romantic, I hoped to find my soulmate and raise a family. Two decades later, I was living my dream. While celebrating my thirty-sixth birthday, I reveled in my loving marriage, busy and fulfilling practice, and three children under six years old.

Weeks later my world went off-script. Excruciating pain led to a diagnosis of indolent lymphoma—a type of cancer with no known cure. Clinical work was not an option, given the debilitating side effects of chemotherapy in that era before effective antiemetics or growth-stimulating factors. I notified my patients by mail that they needed to find temporary care. At home, family and friends helped look after my children. At night while our little ones slept, my husband and I talked endlessly, seesawing mutual support through the distress of my side effects, setbacks, and sadness.

Ten long months later, reopening my office signaled the end of our ordeal. Or so we thought. My return to work lasted only a few months before my office sent out another "Dear Patient" letter, this time announcing the permanent closure of my practice due to my need for more cancer treatment. A brief stint in another doctor's office ended abruptly after my second recurrence. At the time, I didn't know that I'd never again practice hands-on medicine.

Three decades and many courses of treatment later, my lymphoma is in a durable remission. While celebrating my sixty-sixth birthday last year, I reveled in my career as a medical writer—a different but equal passion—and in my newest role as "Grammy." Not long after, I developed localized pain that felt like my original cancer pain. The MRI findings brought tears of relief— "No cancer"—and sadness. The slipped disc responsible for my new pain was not the most worrisome abnormality. The surgeon pointed to other bulging discs and diffuse spinal and hip osteoarthritis. No more jogging or heavy lifting. Daily activities I'd done my entire life without a second thought were now off-limits, as was the joy of picking up my bigger grandchildren for hugs.

My self-image of being athletic dissolved, which triggered a familiar surreal feeling of not recognizing or trusting my body. My expectations and hopes for tomorrow no longer fit my reality. Sobbing to a dear friend, this time I knew my tears would stop soon—and not because arthritis is non–life-threatening or because I'm old. Life-altering loss hurts at any age. The difference was my confidence in the healing power of grief and hope to help me adapt and find what joys remain.

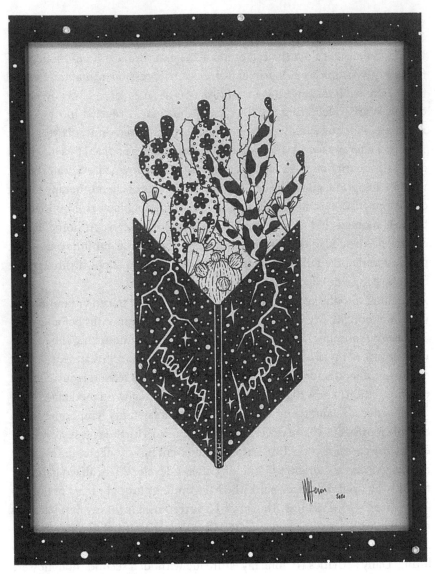

"Healing Hope" by Will Heron

This ink drawing was commissioned in celebration of Dr. Harpham's 66th birthday (October 2020) by Edward Harpham, her husband. Their artist son—a muralist using the professional name, Will Heron—depicts his mother's professional and personal work as rooted in the concept of "Healing Hope." The starry-pattern book doubles as a planter to reference both Dr. Harpham's body of written work and her home. Heron uses his signature Texas cacti to represent the members of their family thriving in harsh conditions while embraced and nurtured by Dr. Harpham's love and compassion. A protective saguaro cactus (her husband) stands behind the three large cacti (their children). The cow-tongue cactus has two blooms, and the cloudy cactus has three blooms. All five flowers (their grandchildren) are infused with the ideals of resilience and healing hope as they grow.

Source: Will Heron, "Healing Hope"

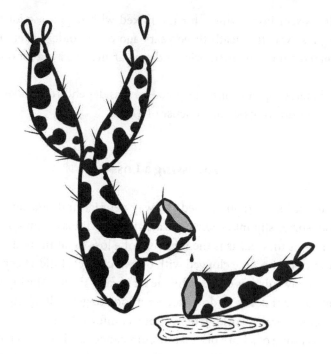

Loss
Source: Will Heron, "Loss"

Understanding Loss

The etymological origin of key words often helps while exploring a complex topic. The Old English term, "los," is of Germanic origin and signifies "destruction."[2] Indeed, every disturbing loss has begun with the destruction of something that mattered to me, changing my perception of or experience in my world.

The object of destruction may be obvious or subtle. The impact may be felt immediately or only after a delay or further destruction.[3] After my first cancer treatments, the premature loss of my menses was clear-cut and unavoidable, while my loss of self-identity was a vague and complex process partly under my control. Decades later, the retirement of my oncologist

[2] Online Etymology Dictionary loss|Origin and meaning. etymonline.com.
[3] Harpham, W. W. (2014). The medicine of grief. *Oncology Times 36*(15), 32 doi:10.1097/01.COT.0000453438.39088.48.

was a bittersweet loss: sadness for me mixed with happiness for him. An agonizing loss was the death three years ago of my older sister, a repository of shared childhood memories and my partner in caring for our elderly mother.

Logic dictates that a healthy response to loss depends on understanding that loss. How does anyone make sense of a loss?

Assessing a Loss

Losses cannot be sized and siloed the way pennies and quarters dropped into a coin sorter slip into their separate slots. Each loss is unique because every person is unique, as is the meaning of a loss to an individual. When my shower drain became clogged with brown clumps, I didn't cry. Sadness about losing my hair was eclipsed by the far greater threat—losing my life—and by my fervent desire to do whatever it took to get well. If anything, the sign of chemotherapy working in my body comforted me.

Each loss is one of a kind because circumstances and people change over time. Prior experiences with a specific loss—and with loss in general—affect hopes and expectations surrounding a new loss. When I lost my second remission, scans showed less disease than when I lost my first remission. Yet I felt more distressed in certain ways because my prognosis was worse and the preceding two and a half years of cancer had worn me out.

Complicating matters, a loss may be linked to other losses. Like the spider's silky web, a tug (a loss) on one strand affects others. A fist through a cobweb may compromise the whole, much as closing my practice felt like a punch to my solar plexus. Hanging up my white coat meant losing the opportunity to use the clinical skills I'd worked years and sacrificed much to develop. It represented "goodbye" to my patients and my office family—people whom I cared about and with whom I'd spent most of my waking hours. Without my routines, I fumbled around at home in unstructured time. The loss of my income sparked worries about my family's financial future. A most painful loss was innocently pointed out by my oldest child while helping me and a few friends stuff envelopes with "Dear Patient" letters. One of the women had started telling a story, saying, "Since Wendy is a doctor. . . ." Seven-year-old Becky interrupted, "Mom *used* to be a doctor."[4]

Distinguishing Insignificant and Significant Losses

The avalanche of losses associated with my illness destroyed my "normal." Categorizing them gave me a toehold in making sense of what was happening. Despite the inherent limitations of such groupings, the exercise provides a useful framework for assessing my response and seeing what more I can do—or what I can do differently—to adjust and move on. To begin, I ask, "How significant is this loss?" The story of my lost keys illustrates how the answer might help.

Cancer-related cognitive impairment caused me to spend hours every week looking for misplaced items. The hit to my self-confidence and loss of time added stress, especially when my searching delayed a family outing, making "my" loss also "theirs." More than once, my husband gently suggested I attach my keys to my pocketbook. The notion of a visible tether reminded me of toddlers' mitten clips, an intolerable loss to my public persona. I resisted . . . and kept dealing with the inconvenience, frustration, stress, and eroded self-esteem associated with repeatedly misplacing my keys. One day I asked myself, "How big a deal is it, really, if an attachment pokes out of my purse?" Stepping back, I saw that loss as insignificant. My unpleasant emotions lessened, and I set off to a hardware store in search of a fun accessory. After a few days, the sight of my neon-pink plastic key coil comforted me, symbolizing my taking control by eliminating a source of distress.[5]

More often, my miscalculations erred on the side of underestimating a blow. That helps explain my wrestling for years with what felt like excessive sadness and frustration about my ongoing need for daily rests. Co-survivors in my support group seemed more accepting of the slower pace. Some even welcomed it, which made me wonder, "What's wrong with me?" Self-doubt and loneliness were exacerbated in social settings each time any mention of

---

[4] Harpham, W. S. (2007) Saving my self. *Oncology Times 29*(17), 34. doi:10.1097/01.COT.00002954 98.33087.3bdoi:10.1097/01.COT.0000295498.33087.3b. https://journals.lww.com/oncology-times/ Fulltext/2007/09100/Saving_My_Self.12.aspx

[5] Harpham, W. S. (2019). Helping patients cope with losing things. *Oncology Times 41*(4), 12. doi:10.1097/01.COT.0000553978.53167.2c.

my fatigue was greeted with bromides such as, "It's a small price . . . you're alive!" and "I wish I could nap every day!"

The turning point was an invitation to discuss the patient experience at a national meeting of the Fatigue Coalition, a group of researchers and clinicians. In my analytical-doctor mind space, I teased apart the tangle of challenges due to fatigue-related losses. Designing graphics for my PowerPoint enabled me to see for the first time the sticky web of thoughts and feelings trapping me, which led to insights on how to resolve my frustration.[6]

That therapeutic writing venture taught me an important lesson: what matters more than *what* I feel is *what I do* with what I feel. Fighting or hiding unpleasant emotions wastes energy and, worse, represents lost opportunity. I do better when I stop and ask myself, "Are my unpleasant emotions the signal of a problem or the response to one?"

Persistent unpleasant emotions sometimes signal a loss I have not yet acknowledged. More often, I know exactly what I've lost but have mistakenly minimized it. While struggling with the loss of my practice and the loss of my stamina, the notion of emotions as a signal prompted me to recalibrate both those losses as "huge," which helped me welcome the next bursts of tears as commensurate grief. Healing grief.

The journey from acknowledgment to acceptance varies. In the example of my resistance to using a key chain, I experienced a few days' lag between identifying the associated loss as "insignificant" and wholeheartedly accepting it. Other times, my rational assessment that a loss is insignificant produces immediate and complete acceptance. End of story. In contrast, the "significant" label invariably marks the opening paragraph of a new chapter because the greater impact poses greater challenges. That categorization helps me manage my expectations, gear up for the work of acceptance and adaptation, and ask for assistance sooner rather than later.

Categorizing Significant Loss

For a significant loss, it sometimes helps to further categorize it as a loss of (1) something, (2) someone, (3) part of my body or mind, or (4) my life.

[6] Harpham, W. S. (1999). Resolving the frustration of fatigue. CA: A Cancer Journal for Clinicians 49(3), 178–189. https://doi.org/10.3322/canjclin.49.3.178.

Broadly, those subdivisions differ in the complexion of my pain, my ability to influence the outcome, my expectations and hopes regarding the future, and my need for guidance and support. Put another way, the subjective experience is different, as are the features and magnitude of the obstacles to finding acceptance and adjusting in healthy ways.

For a loss of some*thing* that matters to me, I'm limited in my ability to change what happened. Whether I've lost my wallet or closed my medical practice, the destruction is done. My power lies in the fact that I am still "me." I can choose to refashion my personal world, whether by replacing the wallet (and its contents) or by finding work in another practice.

The loss of some*one* shares many similarities to the loss of something: I am still "me," with the power to make practical adjustments to the absence of that person. There the similarity ends. Cliché but true, our relationships with others are what matter most in this life. The challenge arises from the loss of all real-time connections through bidirectional physical exchanges of words, gazes, actions, or touch. The severing of those modes of communication redefines those relationships. Whatever one's beliefs about life after death, for the bereaved the experience of those relationships continues in the mind. If I'd normally call a particular friend, I can still feel connected by talking to the spirit of that person and imagining what that friend would say or do. If feeling someone's presence while listening to "our" song or reading an old letter, my experience cannot be shared with that person in the usual ways. I'm comforted by the permanence of our shared past, filled with good moments that nobody can take away. The pain of my grief is lessened by the idea that its intensity reflects the strength of the bond. What gives me hope is my sense that love never dies. The legacies of friends and loved ones can live on, but if—and only if—I work at it. The greatest ways to honor others' memories are by embracing my life, changed as it is without them, and finding ways to feel their love and continue their legacies in life-enhancing ways.

A loss involving my body or mind falls into a different category because the space enveloped by my skin houses "me." If a loss changes my appearance, sensations, or abilities in a way I despise, I can't trade in my body as I did when my new minivan turned out to be a lemon. Power arises from adjusting my perceptions and behaviors in healthy, hopeful ways. If unsure whether a loss is permanent, the notion of creating a "new normal for now" inspires me to make life the best it can be today while holding on to hope for tomorrow. After losing the physical stamina needed for clinical medicine,

I invested heart and soul into my writing and patient advocacy. Those were the best ways to help patients until, if possible, I regained the well-being needed for patient care—a hope kept alive by renewing my medical license year after year.

If I'm feeling powerless while facing the loss of something or someone, I turn to the teaching of psychiatrist and Holocaust survivor Viktor Frankl: "Everything can be taken from a [person] but one thing: the last of the human freedoms—to choose one's attitude in any given set of circumstances."[7] That belief has been a source of inspiration since reading *Man's Search for Meaning* in college.

The fourth category, my own death, involves loss I can only imagine. My thoughts and feelings about this challenge were first shaped by my experiences caring for patients and then by my visits with young support-group friends during their final days. At thirty-nine, I came closer to facing my own mortality while enrolled in a Phase I study of the first monoclonal antibody therapy used to treat cancer. I hoped the treatments might work. As a scientist, I lived with the knowledge that I'd likely die before my eldest child graduated elementary school. Fearing death, I envisioned the loss of all earthly sensations and communications. What tore me up most was the idea of leaving behind everything and everyone I knew and the image of my beloved husband raising our children without me.

Our children are now grown, with their own families. After entering this lasting remission, my time horizon narrowed slowly as the flickering candles on my birthday cakes reflected increasing certainty that most of my life was behind me. My perspective on death shifted suddenly in the spring of my sixty-third year while sitting beside my sister, Debra, through her final hours. Knowing her passing was imminent and that she could still hear us, I tried desperately to find the most comforting and loving last words. I happened to have glanced at her face the moment that she suddenly opened her eyes, saw something that made her smile, and expired. That image seared in my memory, permanently weakening my hardwired denial—and fear—of death.

Loss is part of the human condition. We can't choose many of the losses we face. We can always choose how we respond.

---

[7] Frankl, V. E. (1984). *Man's search for meaning*. Revised and updated (p. 86). New York: Washington Square Press.

Approach to Loss

As both a physician and a cancer survivor, I believe patients play a central role in their survivorship, by which I mean the science and art of making life the best it can be after a diagnosis. To cope with loss, I've turned to the first verse of a version of Reinhold Niebuhr's popular "Serenity Prayer"[8] (also called "The Courage Prayer"), praying for the courage to learn how to recover what's lost, repair or mitigate the loss, or, when possible, replace what's lost. Then I pray for the courage to act on that knowledge, doing what must be done to influence the outcome.

After immutable, irreplaceable loss, I pray for serenity. That word conjures up images of stillness and tranquility. Yet arriving at a place of peaceful acceptance and adaptation usually demands activity and uneasiness. It takes courage and fortitude to do the emotional work, such as cognitive reframing, letting go of beliefs and habits that no longer serve me well, and forgiving myself (or someone else) for an action or inaction that may have caused or exacerbated the loss. Add on the practical challenges of creating a "new normal,"[9] such as learning new ways to do everyday things and practicing new skills until they come more naturally. Depending on the loss, I may need to invest in physical (or other) therapy or counseling—demanding work by any measure.

Grieving After Significant Loss

During a counseling session soon after closing my practice, when I could barely talk through embarrassingly uncontrollable crying, my social worker stated a simple truth: the human response to loss is grief. The matter-of-fact way she said it kept me from ever again seeing my tears as weakness or apologizing for them. These days, whenever I get choked up, I use self-talk, sometimes with a splash of comic relief, "There you go again: being human!"

Along with appreciating the link between loss and grief, I needed to understand what grief entails. After leaving the social worker's office that day,

[8] Niebuhr, R. (n.d.). "Serenity Prayer." The Prayer Foundation. https://www.prayerfoundation.org/dailyoffice/serenity_prayer_full_version.htm.

[9] Harpham, W. S. (2019). Introducing the New Normal for now. *Oncology Times* 41(19),12. doi:10.1097/01.COT.0000586252.40444.88.   https://journals.lww.com/oncology-times/blog/ViewFromtheOtherSideoftheStethoscope/pages/post.aspx?PostID=24

I stopped on the way home to stock up on tissues, determined to get through my grief in world-record time. If elite swimmers could breathe more efficiently, I could grieve more efficiently. Right?

Reality humbled me. The spectrum of my symptoms included otherwise inexplicable irritability, poor appetite, foggy thinking, disrupted sleep, or a vague melancholy while surrounded by smiling, laughing people. At times, I'd enter a situation feeling emotionally prepared for expected triggers, and yet waterworks would surprise me.

Those experiences led me to a second truth: we can only influence—not control—our grief. My influence begins with acknowledging and naming a loss and doing the same for the cascade of secondary losses. Then comes the labor: finding safe spaces and techniques for expressing whatever I am thinking or feeling. Journaling comes naturally but, by itself, is rarely enough. Significant loss often seeks the healing power of witnessing—someone hearing and seeing my emotions in real time and showing compassion without trying to fix it.[10]

Usually, I find sanctuary in the company of a dear friend or my husband, with whom I share everything. Early in my survivorship, though, I turned to professionals to help me work through painful thoughts and feelings, some of which were embarrassing, shameful, selfish, or petty. That degree of emotional nakedness would have been painful for my loved ones and intolerable for me. With professionals, I could let down my guard, knowing they'd sympathize without empathizing and would leave my world once I regained equilibrium.[11]

In workshops and keynote addresses I emphasize, "There is no single 'right' way to grieve, but there are best ways for each person for each loss. People grieve in their own way on their own schedule. Some don't need to cry—and shouldn't be made to think they're supposed to." Then, speaking to attendees who might be denying or suppressing grief, I make fun of myself: "I doubt that anyone here cries as much as I did. If tears cured cancer, I would not have needed chemo." My hope is that presenting myself as Queen Crier helps attendees overcome obstacles to expressing grief.

Those same messages helped me through the first week after my consultation with the back surgeon, when I learned about my spinal arthritis.

[10] Harpham, W. S. (2014). Patient handout: Honoring grief. *Oncology Times 36*(16), 38. doi:10.1097/01.COT.0000453671.96155.fe.

[11] Harpham, W. S. (2016). Social workers on the oncology team. *Oncology Times 38*(22), 32. doi:10.1097/01.COT.0000508622.74027.53.

Each time I added an activity to my "forbidden activities" list, a wave of sadness washed over me. In the middle of the night, when pain made sleep impossible, I remembered the conclusion of my keynote comments: "Having expressed my grief and found ways to adapt, the urge to cry disappeared." Whatever happens with my back pain, today my grief—disruptive emotions that I'm choosing to express without inhibition—is less painful thanks to my hope of adjusting and feeling whole again.

Finding Hope After Significant Loss

Hope is key to dealing with loss in healthy ways. When my prognosis worsened after my second recurrence, people kept insisting, "Wendy, you have to have hope." Unable to turn on "hope" like a light switch, I realized how little I knew about this uniquely human emotion. That launched a quest to learn what it is, how it works, and how patients find hope. Not just any hope, but healing hope—namely, hope that helps patients get good care and live as fully as possible.[12]

Hope works in two ways: motivating me to action or, when there's nothing to do, helping me wait. In my search for healing hope, I began asking myself whether what I'm hoping for motivates me to effective action. If waiting helplessly, I ask whether what I am hoping for is decreasing or increasing my anxiety.

For years after seeing my last patient, my white coat hung in the front of my closet, feeding my belief in the possibility of returning to patient care someday, somehow. Instinctively, I let that hope float in the wings while keeping center stage all actionable hopes, such as of finding meaning and joy in writing. Throughout the subsequent years, hope of continuing my life-long mission of "Helping others through the synergy of science and caring" motivated me to pursue opportunities out of my comfort zone, such as public speaking, survivorship advocacy, and teaching university students.

As for my post-treatment fatigue, for too long I hoped to muscle through the day, which left me irritable and prone to making mistakes. After I finally let go of that and focused instead on hope of respecting limits, I felt better physically and made fewer mistakes.[13] That helped, but it didn't stop the

[12] Harpham, W. S. (2018). *Healing hope: Through and beyond cancer*. Dallas, Texas, New York: Curant House.
[13] Harpham, W. S. (1994). *After cancer: A guide to your new life*. New York: W. W. Norton.

pangs of sadness when I lay down to nap. My ongoing hope for others to sympathize with my struggle was both unrealistic and harmful, increasing my sense of alienation. Peace came with hoping instead for my innermost circle of people to believe me—even if they didn't understand my naptime blues.

Where there is hope, there is life. In every situation, there is always *something* good to hope for.[14] The key is figuring out which hopes help me act and which help me wait. In all cases, I nourish hopes of setting the stage for meaning and joy in life.

Facing Death

The final breath snuffs out all hope. No more opportunities to adapt. No more possibility of finding meaning or joy in this life. My thoughts and feelings about death—including my fears and hopes about my own—have been shaped in large part by my experiences living with a poor long-term prognosis while raising my young children. The heightened uncertainty about my health made parenting more distressing. At the same time, it made it easier by clarifying my purpose: to use whatever time I had to love them and teach them the skills and values that would help them live their best life.

My approach to parenting through cancer was built on a fundamental belief: the greatest gift we can give our children is not protection from the world, but the confidence and tools to cope and grow with all that life offers.[15] Child-friendly mantras intended to help my children helped me. Some promoted acceptance, such as *Life is not fair*, and *Things can go wrong even when I do everything right*. Others fostered hope and a sense of empowerment, such as *Life is good, even when it's not what we wanted or expected*, and *In every situation we can strive to make life the best it can be*. Finally, with hope of countering the mystique of the independent lone wolf, I'd repeat what became a mantra: *Asking for help is a sign of strength*.

My confidence in my approach grew as I watched my children blossom despite my many absences and their cancelled birthday parties. Cancer recurrences pushed me to use everyday opportunities to keep talking about the circle of life. In response to their questions, I searched for answers that

---

[14] Harpham. Patient handout: Healing hope.
[15] Harpham, W. S. (1997). *When a parent has cancer: A guide to caring for your children*. New York: HarperCollins.

would nurture realistic hope of my recovery while reassuring them they'd be cared for and happy, whatever happened with me.

One evening during our routine bedtime chat, my eldest child asked whether I would die. As planned and practiced in anticipation of that moment, I acknowledged that, yes, I would die someday . . . and might die of cancer. In the same breath that I told her she'd feel sad, I asserted she wouldn't always feel that sad. She'd feel happy again. Taking her hands in mine, I promised she'd feel my love whenever she wanted to. After expressing my great hope of growing old, I shifted to short-term actionable hope by asking for ideas on how to make the next day the best it could be. My good-night kiss on her forehead came with a guarantee: "You will always feel my love." Becky fell asleep easily that night. The task done, I went to my bedroom, called a friend, and wept, feeling more hopeful about my children and indescribably sad for me.

Throughout the years when my life was most in danger, my attention was focused on minimizing the negative impact on my children if I should die and not on preparing myself or what it would mean for me. Ironically, I seriously imagined my own death for the first time while my health was relatively stable and I was supporting my sister, Debra, through her final illness.

Once again, my professional experiences gave me confidence in my ability to guide and support a loved one, with a critical difference: "sister" mode was the antithesis of "mother" mode. My approach with my children was driven by my desire to instill my values for what I expected to be their long lives. With my sister, I strained to keep my beliefs and opinions to myself, even when discussing options that I had faced as a patient. My goal was to help Debra work her way to informed decisions in keeping with *her* values, not mine. She reassured me I was succeeding the day she snapped, "You can stop saying that! I know it's my decision and you'll support whatever I decide."

Throughout our many difficult conversations, I expressed my sympathy, a distinctly human emotion binding people together with a sense of shared feelings. The paradox of sympathy is that I cannot possibly feel or know the totality of another's experience, no matter how extensive our conversations and sincere my efforts to imagine it. When Debra asked, "What should I do?" and "Wendy, what would you do?" I responded as I had over the years to other patients with whom I'd sympathized: "Only you can know what's best for you. As for what I'd do if it were me, I cannot know without being in the situation." I assured her I could still help, just as I could help patients manage their insulin even though I'd never had diabetes.

Sympathy benefitted us both by enabling me to share in my sister's experience and reach across the divide with compassion. My sympathy as a co-survivor made most of our conversations more fruitful. My sympathy as a sister helped in different ways but sometimes intensified the challenge for me. Determined to keep the conversation centered on her and her needs, I tried to maintain my composure until after I hung up. Sometimes I failed. When her voice cracked, mine cracked, too. When she responded with gasping grief, I could barely breathe, let alone talk.

Four years into Debra's illness, her suffering kept increasing, with shorter respites. I broached the option of stopping treatment, prepared to share facts and insights I'd articulated in my writings, oncology Grand Rounds presentations, and conversations with other patients.[16,17,18,19,20,21] Yet during our first discussion of pros and cons, I hesitated, dreading the task. Was I ready to let go of my own hope that further treatment would save her? Reluctantly, I proceeded to explain the benefits of hospice. Uttering the familiar phrases proved far more onerous than I knew possible—and I was aware my burden was light compared to my sister's. After she died the following spring, my grief was such that I could not understand why our language doesn't have a unique word for the pain of surviving a sibling.

Losing Debra didn't teach me that I'd die one day; it helped me know it in a new way. Her death didn't alter my faith; it changed how I experience my faith, especially in moments when I sense her spirit, such as while caring for our mother. Losing my sister changed my understanding of what it means to lose a loved one. It reinforced my belief that I cannot imagine what I will feel

[16] Harpham, W. S. (2011). Stopping time. *Oncology Times 33*(13), 37. doi:10.1097/01.COT.0000400084.74566.c1.   https://journals.lww.com/oncology-times/Fulltext/2011/07100/VIEW_FROM_THE_OTHER_SIDE_OF_THE_STETHOSCOPE_.13.aspx

[17] Harpham, W. S. (2011). Helpful, hopeful handout when stopping chemotherapy. *Oncology Times 33*(14), 20. doi:10.1097/01.COT.0000403400.42210.d1. https://journals.lww.com/oncology-times/Fulltext/2010/05100/VIEW_FROM_THE_OTHER_SIDE_OF_THE_STETHOSCOPE__A.13.aspx

[18] Harpham, W. S. (2018). Patient handout: Understanding promising unproven therapies. *Oncology Times 40*(17), 28. doi:10.1097/01.COT.0000546193.07744.98. https://journals.lww.com/oncology-times/Fulltext/2018/09050/Patient_Handout__Understanding_Promising_Unproven.20.aspx

[19] Harpham, W. S. (2018). To try or not to try. *Oncology Times 40*(13), 16. doi:10.1097/01.COT.0000542463.45794.c2. https://journals.lww.com/oncology-times/Fulltext/2018/07050/To_Try_or_Not_to_Try.19.aspx

[20] Harpham, W. S. (2018). Soliloquy on a life-and-death decision. *Oncology Times 40*(15), 16–17. doi:10.1097/01.COT.0000544353.31238.a9.   https://journals.lww.com/oncology-times/Fulltext/2018/08050/Soliloquy_on_a_Life_and_Death_Decision.24.aspx

[21] Harpham, W. S. (2019). Patients' hope for a miracle. *Oncology Times 41*(1), 16. doi:10.1097/01.COT.0000552850.91141.07.   https://journals.lww.com/oncology-times/Fulltext/2019/01050/Patients__Hope_for_a_Miracle.23.aspx

or how I'll respond when my time comes—and that I don't need to know. The best ways to honor the memory of those I've lost are by treasuring what time I have, asking for whatever help I need to make my days the best they can be, and by trusting that when my time comes I'll face my end with grace.

At the end of January 2022, a diagnosis of aplastic anemia fractured my world and brought me the closest I've come to facing my mortality. Lessons learned about doing loss kept me from succumbing to a sickening sense of doom. Determined to get through the worst grief and adjust to my new reality, I sought wisdom and strength in a prayer: *Please don't let me die before I die.* Fulfilling that prayer depended on my

- *Putting sympathy on a shelf.* Feeling my loved ones' distress and envisioning them grieving after I die only made things worse now for me and for them.
- *Not indulging in visions of progressive illness and death.* I'll deal with those challenges when my time comes—and not a moment sooner.
- *Finding hopes for today and for tomorrow.* There is always something good to hope for.

This latest illness forced me to see anew and accept more completely that earthly life is temporary. It comforts me knowing that passing away is peaceful, a fact learned from the literature and convincingly illustrated by my sister's smile. As for wrestling with mortality, that's necessarily solitary. Through fear and with faith, I'll give it my best. Meanwhile, maternal love inspires me to model for my children and grandchildren how grieving and hoping line the path to finding happiness after loss. In my never-ending striving to make life the best it can be, I'm living my best life today, tomorrow, and every day.

Living After Loss

For the rest of my life, I'll keep doing loss as best I can. Sometimes with tears. Often with the sympathy and support of others. Always by honoring my grief and finding hope. Loss is a great teacher, enabling all of us to know both the fragility and the hopes of life, and with that knowledge to live most fully.

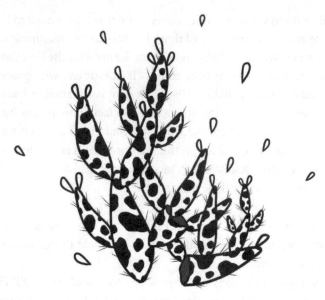

Living after Loss
Source: Will Heron, "Living after Loss"

About the Author

Wendy S. Harpham, MD, FACP, is a doctor of internal medicine and thirty-one-year cancer survivor. Forced by illness to retire from patient care nine years after opening her solo practice, she turned to writing, speaking, and patient advocacy. She authored two textbook chapters and eight books on survivorship, including two children's books and one for clinicians. Since 2005, she has written an award-winning column in *Oncology Times*. Her work addresses common challenges of survivorship, such as managing uncertainty, coping with fatigue, raising children while ill, and finding healing hope—namely, hope that helps patients get good care and live as fully as possible. Dr. Harpham has served as a consultant or patient advocate on local and national advisory committees and survivorship working groups. An adjunct professor at the University of Texas at Dallas from 2011 through 2021, Dr. Harpham taught and mentored pre-health undergraduates. The American College of Physicians honored her with the 2018 Nicholas E. Davies Memorial Award for Scholarly Activities in the Medical Humanities. The 2000 Governor's Award for Health led to her induction into the Texas Women's Hall of Fame.

Suggested Resources

Books

Fink, J. (2012). *When you lose someone you love*. Morton Grove, Illinois: Publications International Limited.

Puri, S. (2019). *That good night*. New York: Viking.

Kalanithi, P. (2016). *When breath becomes air*. New York: Random House.

Articles

Harpham, Wendy S. (2014). The medicine of grief. *Oncology Times 36*(15), 32. https:// journals.lww.com/oncology-times/Fulltext/2014/08100/View_from_the_Other_S ide_of_the_Stethoscope__The.25.aspx

Harpham, Wendy S. (2014). Patient handout: Honoring grief. *Oncology Times 36*(16), 38. https://tinyurl.com/OTHonoringGrief

3

"Will You Take Me In?"

A Story of Loss, Restoration, and Success

Damon Madison

Waiting for My Father at School

When I was in first grade, my elementary school had a Father–Student Day. I fantasized that my father was going to attend. He never communicated to me that he would, but I had hope he knew about it and would surprise me. He never made it. I was devastated and embarrassed because all the other students had their fathers. After school, I sat on the schoolhouse stoop, waiting, hoping he would show up. The teacher parking lot began to empty. A kind teacher came up to me and asked, "Damon, are you ok? Is your parent coming?" "Yes," I lied. "Ok, get home safe," she replied and went on her way.

I waited two hours for my father not to show up.

I held my head down and started crying, thinking how ridiculous am I to have such a dream. I do not know why I thought he would come. I walked home, again disappointed. I knew very little about my father. I never met him. My mother would often tell me, "Your father is a deadbeat." We had no contact information, and he provided no support, financial or otherwise. Not knowing my father or having any contact with him made me feel rejected, neglected, and unloved. My friends had their fathers; why didn't I have mine? I could only imagine what a father's love would be like, and I longed for it.

The loss of my father was only the beginning. I wish I could say this was the worst loss I experienced in my life, but the worst was yet to come.

My Family

I grew up from very humble beginnings in the small town of South Bend, Indiana. My mother Iris was a beautiful African American woman, five-foot-ten in stature, with a slender body and long wavy hair. She had a contagious laugh that made anyone around her smile. I admired my mother's confident, strong demeanor. Up until I turned eight years old, Iris, then a single mom of six, held several jobs. I particularly remember when she was a school bus driver. I was proud of her because she enjoyed that job and was able to buy necessities for the household. She had no shortage of love, attention, hugs, kisses, or positive affirmations for my siblings and me. "Good job," she would tell us. "You do everything well." These were happy times.

My siblings and I were close, due largely to my mother's constant reinforcement around the importance of family. "Other people will let you down," she would tell us. At the time, I had three older and two younger siblings. We had each other's backs. We shared food, clothes and helped each other stay on top of our schoolwork. I felt safe and cared for in my home. Suddenly, at the age of eight, all of this changed, and my life would never be the same again.

Where Did My Mother Go?

When I was eight years old, my mother met my stepfather Jerry. Jerry was a 6-foot, 250-pound husky, intimidating man with dark ashy skin that constantly needed a coat of lotion. He was gluttonous, never shared any of his food, and could not keep a job. He had a foul mouth that spewed curse words and insults. He verbally abused my mother in front of us, calling her "bitch" and "stupid." He did not deserve my mother or her love, but, somehow, he had both.

My stepfather's cruel comments and behavior made me angry, not only at him but at my mother for tolerating it. I would think and agonize over how I might protect her, but due to my age and his size, I could not shield her from him. I felt powerless, as if I was in a sealed jar, screaming for help but no one could hear me.

Almost immediately after meeting Jerry, my mother's behavior changed. The time, love and affection once showered on my siblings and me were now given solely to Jerry. Gone were the positive affirmations. Gone was the emphasis on family. Worse still, my mother's behavior increasingly mirrored Jerry's. She stopped working. She barked orders without concern or interest for our well-being. No matter how hard we tried, we could not reach her, the mother we once knew, the mother who once protected us. And I desperately needed protection.

One afternoon, my siblings and I were playing hide-and-go-seek when my stepfather became angry because I was running in the house. He suddenly and without warning grabbed me by the throat and choked me. My siblings were shocked and scared and ran screaming to our mother. She got angry at him, but also with us. She slapped my siblings and me and told us never to run in the house again. She then packed my stepfather's belongings and threw him out of the house. I was relieved! I thought my mother must truly love me if she sent Jerry away. Finally, I felt safe again, protected and cared for.

But one month later, Jerry moved back in. I was baffled and enraged. How could my mother allow him back into our home and our lives? I felt rejected by my mother. I had lost my mother's love again. My sense of safety and well-being evaporated. I lost my appetite and quite a bit of weight. The anguish and fear that at any moment I would be slapped by Jerry's giant fat hand kept me up at night. I kept a knife under my pillow to protect myself.

Within a few months of his return, the beatings resumed. Jerry would strike me with curtain rods, extension cords, tree switches, belts, hairbrushes, skillets. My skin was a patchwork of bruises, cuts, contusions. Yet my mother did not intercede. There were times when the abuse was so violent, I needed medical attention. Other times, my mother and Jerry did not allow me to receive any medical attention to avoid child abuse charges, losing their children, or going to jail.

The beatings only got worse. Until one day, when I was eleven years old, Jerry ordered me to bend over and hold my ankles so he could beat me with a 2 × 4 wooden plank. I was so sick, tired, and demoralized by being physically and emotionally abused. I remember thinking to myself, "What do I have to lose? If he kills me, at least I wouldn't endure this torture anymore." I did not bend over. Rather, I told Jerry, "I am moving out of the house and will no longer take any of your abuse." This was the first time I did not obey his demands. Jerry sat on the chair, leaned the plank between his legs, and said, "You are not going anywhere." He stood up. I stood my ground. What came next surprised me. "You stood up to me," Jerry said. "You will be very successful one day." And he left the room. For the first time in my life, I allowed myself to feel liberated and empowered. I had the strength to stand up to his abuse. My fear of Jerry decreased significantly. I no longer looked at him as a potential father-figure, but as an *abuser*.

"Get Your Ass Out There and Don't Come Home Without Money"

Within three years after Jerry came into our home, he and my mother, in rapid succession, had three children. They did not experience the abuse I did because they were my stepfather's biological children. With nine people now living in the house, it was overcrowded and uncomfortable, with seldom enough food to go around. For the first time in my life, I experienced hunger. When there was no food in the house—and I mean no food—I scrounged up what I could. I would make sugar and butter sandwiches for breakfast, lunch, *and* dinner. I added hot water to chicken broth. Most nights, I went to bed starving. It was the worst feeling. I was angry and scared. There was nothing for me to do but pray for food, drink water, and secretly cry myself to sleep.

My mother and Jerry did nothing to ease our hunger. They stayed home, watched their television stories, and did not make any effort to gain employment. Rather, they demanded that I be the one to work for food to feed the entire family. "Get your ass out there and don't come home without money," my mother and Jerry would scream at me. I was terrified that if I didn't bring home money, they would beat me. I know this is hard to believe.

I did whatever I could to make money, given my young age. Simultaneously, I had a *Tribune* paper route, mowed lawns, raked leaves, shoveled snow, and did odd jobs for the neighbors. When I returned home, my mother would take 100% of the money I earned. I was left with nothing but my sadness and rage. From this I learned that I could not be honest if I wanted to survive. I began to lie about how much money I made that day. My mother (and Jerry) would only get 90% of what I made. Lying was, at least initially, very hard for me to do and had negative implications for my personal integrity. I also knew that it was a serious sin. I felt so trapped.

In addition to working multiple jobs, my mother and Jerry singled me out to care for their three young kids. My parents were home all day, unemployed, yet I was forced to care for their kids day and night. I changed their diapers, fed, and bathed them. At night, my mother would roll the bassinet into my room. "But I have school in the morning," I would tell her. "I don't care," she replied. I would have to do the baby's middle-of-the-night feedings, which meant waking up at 3 A.M., walking downstairs, opening the can of formula, boiling water to warm the formula, testing the formula on my wrist to make sure it wasn't too hot, then back upstairs to feed her and rock her to sleep. *I was twelve years old.*

My parents all too often forced me to stay home from school to take care of their kids. I was the only child kept home from school. One year, I missed three consecutive months of elementary school. When I expressed concern to my parents about falling behind, they asked my older brother Ron to collect my assignments from the teachers. I had to teach it all to myself. I felt so trapped and was filled with so much resentment toward my parents for prohibiting me from furthering my education. Despite all this, I was extremely successful. I was surprised by my ability to understand new concepts by reading alone, without being in class. I maintained straight A's and made Honor Roll. This experience gave me hope and a sense of accomplishment in a life where I was only told: "you are no good and selfish."

At times, it was as if I was the only parent in the home. I did not know what it was to have a childhood. I was unable to participate in the fun outdoor activities with my peers as I was always caring for the kids, doing household chores, or working. I was demoralized, humiliated, and exhausted. I could not control the feeling and accept the reality that my childhood had been stolen by the very people who were supposed to protect it.

The Last Beating and Beating the Odds

When I was fourteen years old, I was putting one of Jerry's kids down for her nap. She was fussy, and, in frustration, I raised my voice to her. Jerry heard. "Come here," he barked. Without warning, he punched me hard in the chest, knocking the wind out of me. The unexpected blow was so strong, I flew across the room and slammed into the wall. It really hurt but for some reason the humiliation was worse. I felt a rage burning inside of me like I had never felt before. I went into an altered state. I could only think of one thing: How can I destroy this beast of a man? As I fell to the floor, I scanned the room for a weapon to use against him. My eyes caught a screwdriver on the desk. I wanted to stab him in the head. I jumped up, grabbed the screwdriver, and lunged at him, but he ducked out of the way, and the screwdriver got stuck deep into the woodwork. I dangled over the ground in panic, trying to unwedge the screwdriver from the wall so I could finish the job. I was blind with rage and lost all control. I wanted to hurt him for the many years he hurt me, my Mom, and my siblings. My mother began screaming, "Stop, stop, stop!" My mother's voice snapped me out of my rage. My stepfather was at the edge of his bed, on his knees, pleading with me to stop. I heard my mother's all-too-familiar, empty refrain, "This will never happen again." I had enough. I heard a voice, me and not me, screaming: "I am done with this." I knew I needed to leave. If I didn't, either I was going to die, or they were going to die. But where and how? I had enough, but I also had nothing and nowhere to go.

God on My Side

As the abuse became more psychologically and physically extreme, I increasingly thought of ways to escape. Fortunately, my mother still took us to church every Sunday. Church was a true refuge for me. Attending weekly services taught me the value of prayer, which, in turn, provided me an outlet to safely share my frustrations, hopes, and dreams. I needed to try to trust God because I had no one else to believe in. I would rather put my trust in someone that I could not see because the people I *could* see only failed me. I had no father or mother to protect me from the abuse. I would pray to God to remove me from it. Sunday services were the only times I felt at peace. It was my faith that helped me cope with the abuse I suffered at the hands of those who were supposed to be my biggest protectors and champions. When all is said and done, my prayers have always been answered. It was also my faith that led me to my true protectors and champions, Kathy and Mrs. Campbell.

Shelter from the Storm: Kathy and Mrs. Campbell

My neighbor Kathy was a fifty-year-old Caucasian woman with blond hair and fair skin. She dressed to impress, with designer clothes, and manicured nails. She would decorate her nails according to each holiday throughout the year. She had no children and was never married. Kathy was one of my regular customers. I raked her leaves, mowed her lawn, and shoveled her snow.

I felt safe with Kathy. I told her about the abuse. One day she asked me, "Damon, do you want to go to college?" "Yes, I want that very much," I replied. "You are not going to college if you stay in that house." I told her I was ready to leave. Kathy agreed to help me. She researched ways in which I might legally leave my home. I was just fifteen years old. I would get to go to college and graduate school as well. I would thrive in that supportive learning environment after getting off to a rough start, being away from home. It was determined that my best bet to be removed from the home was to be taken in by a church elder, Mrs. Campbell.

Mrs. Campbell was also Caucasian. She had beautiful, fair skin, rosy, red cheeks, and brunette hair. She and her husband lived alone as their two kids had gone off to college. Although they were open to the idea, interracial co-habitation in the Midwest was not encouraged. In fact, it was well-known back then that we had to be very careful about where we went and how we interacted. The Ku Klux Klan was very active in Indiana, particularly in our area, and struck fear into blacks (for merely being black) and whites who did not share their racist views. The KKK was very real and dangerous. Oddly, despite how close we grew, we did not openly talk about race, but it was a reality in our lives. There was one time when Mr. Campbell, a quiet and accepting gentleman, said to me: "Damon you made me realize that not all black people are the same." I think it took a lot of courage for him to admit this perspective, and although it made me feel uncomfortable, it helped to me to understand his thought process. Upon reflection, I only now realize what risks Kathy and the Campbells took on my behalf.

One Sunday, during a freezing blizzard in South Bend, I was walking home from the grocery store. It was a seven-mile walk, and I was about halfway home. I was carrying five grocery bags and was without winter gloves. I will never forget barely seeing Mrs. Campbell's burgundy minivan through squinted eyes. She pulled up next to me and rolled down the passenger window. "Damon, is that you?" I am not even sure how she recognized me as the gusting winds and deluge of snow blocked almost all visibility. "Yes, Mrs. Campbell, it's me." "Get in this van," she told me, and, without a thought, I opened the minivan door, put the groceries on the floor, and jumped into the passenger seat. The minivan was warm, and I sighed in relief. I was able to thaw out my frozen hands, which had deep blue welts on them from the plastic bag handles. I was excited to see Mrs. Campbell, but also angry and embarrassed that my parents, once again, had put me in a dangerous situation. The anger gave me the courage to speak up.

"Mrs. Campbell, will you take me in?" "Absolutely, I will take you in." Mrs. Campbell understood my desperate situation due to her good perception and caring personality. It was sad to tell my Mom I was leaving the family. She did not take it well. She said, "The grass isn't greener on the other side." I said, "Well, it's burnt up over here." This was both a wonderful and depressing time for me.

I could not know then that "Damon, is that you?" would change my life forever. Yes, that was me, but that was not the man I was becoming! Kathy worked with an attorney to officially make me an orphan of the state. Mr. and Mrs. Campbell then became my legal guardians. I was fifteen years old and finally free.

I will never forget the very first morning I awoke in my new home with Mr. and Mrs. Campbell. No one asked me for water. No one asked me for food. No one asked me for *anything*. It was quiet. It felt amazing. I continued to work, and, when I came home, I handed my paycheck over to Mrs. Campbell. "Sweetheart," as she always called me, "that is your check. You earned it. You need to save it."

Every Sunday after church service, Mr. and Mrs. Campbell would invite the pastor and congregants over for lunch. Mrs. Campbell made the best fried chicken in the whole wide world. "What do you need help with?" I would ask her. "Nothing, you go sit down and relax." When they realized I was allergic to their two dogs, they kept the dogs outside. For the first time in a very long while, I felt seen as a person by an adult. I did not have to look over my shoulder, wondering when someone was going to hit me. They provided sincere love without requesting anything in return. I did not know, until then, that this alternative world even existed! Mrs. Campbell loved me, without any hidden agenda. She wanted me to have all the opportunities life has to offer. For the first time in my life, I felt safe. This was new for me and very scary. All these years later Mrs. Campbell remains my touchstone. Just last week (August 2021), I received this text message from her: "Love you Sweetheart and hope all is going good with you. Thinking of you often. I love you with all my heart, always."

The Reckoning

Given my grades and motivation (and prayer), I got scholarships to go to college. The reckoning I will now share with you came at college and relates to my shame at being dirt poor and coming from such a dysfunctional family. I tried to cope by lying about my past. Earlier on, Kathy would tell me "the lies will catch up to you someday." I have had to unlearn my lie and embrace my past, but at that time I was not able to hear her wise words yet. At college, the nightmares about Jerry were so real, unrelenting and demanded to be heard. Given my faith, not being honest was quite guilt-provoking.

Altering the facts about my disturbing past was an attempt to protect myself from re-experiencing the sense of loss and desperation that was almost always crushing my shoulders. I was in constant fear that I would somehow be sucked backed into my childhood, trapped and powerless. As had happened before in my life, I received help from a deeply caring and competent college counselor who helped me to accept the unvarnished reality of my past and, for the first time, confront my rage at my parents. This was really hard going, especially when the counselor asked me: "Do you wish your parents were dead?" The nightmares are gone.

"I Ache for That Damon"

Despite my positive attitude in life and my genuine affinity for connecting with people, my childhood experiences continue to impact my personal life. It is very difficult for me to fully love or trust people. I would love to get married and have children. I would love to find someone with whom I can exhale, to catch me when I fall. But when I do begin to get close, I am overtaken by fear, fear of being hurt, fear of being betrayed. If my mother can betray me, anyone can. I find myself cutting the person off before they burn me. I see Jerry—and also, sadly, my own father and mother and their neglectful and disloyal traits. I am always waiting for the next unprotected punch to my chest.

The sadness and helplessness I have experienced in my life has motivated me to be successful and gain financial freedom. I have an abnormal level of ambition. I am relentless in how hard I push myself. I cannot and will not depend on anyone to take care of me. I can only trust myself. Everything is on my shoulders. I have to carry the brunt. The more success I have, the more capable I am to do this. I've never known what it's like to call someone father. I've never known what it's like to have the security of going home to my parents. I have worked hard to create a back-up plan for my back-up plan.

I have worked in the pharmaceutical industry for twenty years and have successfully delivered $4.7 billion dollars in sales throughout my career. I have a BA and an MBA. I have held multiple leadership roles and have received many awards for excellence. Yet, despite my professional success, I live in constant fear of losing what I have, of it slipping out of my hands. I know what it is like to live without, to go hungry in the richest country in the world, to have to always be conscious that I am black in a world where race really matters.

As I write this, I think about my much younger self. I ache for that Damon. I wish I could be there for him now. I still feel the pain of what he went through. It motivates me to pay it forward. My friends get to benefit from anything I have. I am supporting my niece financially so she can attend college. I have even looked out for Jerry's kids, as I promised my Mom I would do on her deathbed.

Independence Day

It is Independence Day, July 4, 2020, twenty-five years after I climbed into that burgundy minivan. I am sitting on the patio of my home in Baldwin Hills, California, in a section known to locals as "the Hill." I can see hundreds of fireworks displays across the night sky. I think back to when I first moved to Los Angeles, just over twenty years ago. I knew no one. I had no friends. I had no social or professional network. I had nothing. It had always been my dream to one day live in Baldwin Hills, an affluent African American community in Los Angeles. It is hard to get up on the Hill. Homes are coveted and rarely sold.

When I share my story with friends, they are mystified. "Damon, you are not supposed to be here!" They see my professional success, my home, my positive attitude, and assume I must have come from means, or loving parents, or great schools. If I was my younger self, I wouldn't have corrected them.

Some days are easier than others. I think back to what my Mom told me on her deathbed: "Be specific in your prayers Damon, I prayed for a husband, but I did not pray for a husband who would love my kids. Don't change who you are as a thoughtful person." I think of where I came from and what I prayed for. Then I look down at my phone: there is a text from Mrs. Campbell: "Think of you often and pray for you! Love you always."

I sit on the patio of the home I bought myself on the Hill, and I think back to that first-grader, sitting on the stoop of his school, staring at an empty sidewalk. Now, I am looking out at a sweeping view of the greater Los Angeles skyline: the lights of the downtown skyscrapers, the iconic Hollywood Sign, the Griffith Park Observatory, Beverly Hills, Century City, Westwood, and a front row seat to watch airplanes take off into the sky. A much wider, once unimaginable view of the world.

I look out at the stars, and I give grace to God, who has always been my North Star.

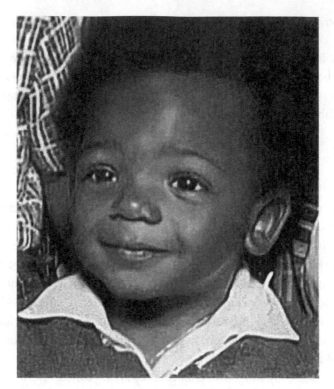

Author, circa age 5

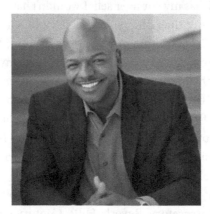

Author, 2021

About the Author

Damon Madison, EMBA, is currently the Head of Inclusion and Diversity for the US Oncology Business Unit working to embed Inclusion & Diversity into the organization's culture. Additionally, Damon is the Senior National Oncology Account Director partnering with strategic accounts where he leads the strategic account engagement with Large Health Systems to advance shared business priorities and advance patient care. This includes portfolio and product communication, ensuring formulary access, and pathway inclusion.

Damon has been recognized with the Circle of Excellence Award within the pharmaceutical industry for his leadership, accomplishments, and strong performance. He has more than twenty-one years of industry experience in a variety of roles, advancing responsibility and experience. Additional leadership experience includes Portfolio Franchise Head, Director of Marketing, Oncology Market Access Director, and Head of Franchise training and sales.

Damon received his bachelor of arts from Ball State University in Muncie, Indiana, and an executive MBA from Pepperdine University in Los Angeles, California.

4

Losing Them

Amy N. Ship

My husband Rob and I have counted six families together, six lives: life as a married couple before children; life with Ari, our first born; life with Ari and Jeremy; life with just Jeremy; life with Jeremy and Jonah; and then life with just Jonah.

At my wedding, looking out over family and friends who had brought me to that day and at the wonderful, witty, kind man I'd just married, I spoke of my charmed life, documenting the gift of ease that my immigrant grandparents had given me through their sacrifices. My paternal great-grandfather abandoned his country, work, and home to give his family a new start. His daughter—my grandmother—hid in an oven to avoid the Cossacks. If it were a novel, my words would have been ironically prescient, the verbal equivalent of Chekov's famous gun. For, twenty-three years later, I write as the mother of three sons, but the "keeper," as it were, of only one—two born profoundly disabled, both now dead, one in 2006 at age four and a half, the other, in 2014, age ten. I look back on myself then, young and filled with hope, never imagining the losses that I'd survive. There is no way I could have predicted or anticipated the loss of even one child, let alone two.

My first son, Ari, was born healthy, failed to achieve developmental milestones, and was ultimately found to have absent white matter—the tissue that allows us to function—in his brain. The words there are intentional, as I'm unable to write "diagnosed." No one was ever diagnosed with anything. Early on, in fact, the words used were "global developmental delay." This is not a diagnosis per se—a name for the disease process—but rather a descriptive term used in medicine when there are no more precise words. And it's also a bit of a lie and, ultimately, felt to me to be a scam, as it suggested that things might improve, that all the doctors could name was a delay. But it's not a delay. It's a fundamental breakdown. There's no catch-up.

So, although physically perfect and quite beautiful, with deep-set brown eyes and a winning smile, Ari wasn't a normal child. Again, I have to choose my words with care. In the twenty-first century, we avoid labeling children as "normal" or "not normal," and appropriately so. But defining your child as "not typically developing" doesn't capture that things were fundamentally wrong. As the years went by, Ari's delays didn't really progress, but neither did they regress. We enrolled him in all the programs we could, and therapists and educators coaxed him along, and he went to an inclusive preschool. And Rob and I did what everyone in the world must do when their lives don't un-roll as expected: we cried and railed and got angry and got sad and then fig-ured out how to go forward.

* * *

Although my second pregnancy lacked the sweet innocence of my first, all went well. Like his brother, Jeremy was a beautiful child. Curly haired and dimpled, Jeremy was as sweet as Ari, but sillier. With Ari, I had been a first-time mother, so every component of concern I raised was met with reassurances until there was clear data—in his case poor growth in his head circumference—that confirmed my fears. With Jeremy, I knew that things were wrong much earlier, by the time he was six weeks old. But once he was a year old, the proof was evident on his MRI, in black and white, as it were. And the findings were worse—less white matter than Ari had; more severe, still unnamable, disease.

Rob and I remember our exact geographic location for each time we re-ceived a call from our pediatrician with the results of an MRI. Although we couldn't have ever imagined on those occasions that we'd ultimately experi-ence it, each call felt like the announcement of a death. Each report was an assault, flinging us into a new, dark, terrifying space. We felt the impact of the news physically and hung on each other in tears and shock. But there was none of the support or ritual that comes with a death. Although the word spread through our community and our friends came to know, none fully understood the depth of our devastation, the profundity of our loss.

And, except for with each other, we couldn't speak of it. When your chil-dren are alive, you cannot even whisper that you've lost them. At best this feels like sacrilege, at worst, prophetic. And yet, each MRI was a pronounce-ment. Each confirmed what had previously only been a thought, a hunch, a fear. Seeing that your son's brain is fundamentally lacking is as much a diag-nosis as one can require; it's graphic proof that something is wrong.

* * *

We had moved from our small apartment to the house that we imagined growing old in three weeks before Jeremy was born. We bought the house on an arc of hope: here was the home in which we'd raise Ari and his assumed-to-be-healthy brother; here was a new chapter in our lives. When we found what looked to me to be a story-book brick house with an extra bedroom and full bath downstairs, we made a bid. It would be a new start, a good one.

I don't remember much of the day-to-day in the years after we moved—the years when both Ari and Jeremy were alive and I was the mother to two sons with special needs. What I remember are the emotions—a sadness and sense of isolation so large that I couldn't share it with anyone. So many journal entries were pleas for help, for relief, for an "out," or expressions of despair. We had no local family, so no one to call for relief. Our friends were caring but had families of their own and never, I think, fully understood the intensity of the chronic challenges we were facing. I couldn't bring myself to tell those who loved me how miserable I was as I knew there was nothing they could say to make it better. And so, I'd hang up the phone yet more despondent, feeling yet more alone.

Everything was hard. Everything. It was like having twin babies, except ones that were much heavier. And it was like *Groundhog Day*: they never grew up, it never got easier. The physical and practical details were crushing. The work was unending: neither could walk, talk, poop, pee, or eat independently. Everything had to be done for them, all the time, always, every day, every night, everywhere. There was no "normal." And there was no reprieve. In fact, in the quiet moments, especially at night in bed, I'd lie awake terrified about the future. How would I manage when they were older and bigger and heavier? How would I manage at all?

I had lost touch with an old friend and reconnected a few months before Ari's death, so I have a document of some of the woes from my email to her. "The time that I devote to coordinating their care or making arrangements or investigating things or goading on those who are trying to help us or taking the boys to appointments is absurd. In the next six weeks, I have appointments for both in gastroenterology, nutrition, endocrine, rehabilitation, general check-up, blood tests, Botox for Ari, orthopedist, developmental educator, and several meetings for Ari's school plan." And all this time, I was working full-time as a primary care physician, teaching and seeing patients and writing. It was impossible to keep on top of everything, and work was unforgiving. I met with my Division Chief to ask that an accommodation be made if I needed to be absent to go to medical appointments. "So, you're asking to be treated as a special case? We can't do that."

In addition to the visits for care, Rob and I went on a mission to find the cause of our sons' brain abnormalities. We didn't care for a diagnosis per se, but rather because a diagnosis might mean a treatment or a cure. It had the capacity to end our nightmare. Alone and together, we spent hours on the internet. The number of unique, rare, inherited disorders is large; for months, we went from disease to disease, perpetually thinking we were about to crack the code. Both Ari and Jeremy's MRIs showed absent white matter in the brain. The umbrella term for this descriptive finding is "leukodystrophy." We read about the seventeen different kinds of leukodystrophies then known and tried to match Ari's characteristics with those described. But babies with his findings were described as dying in infancy, and Ari was three and (relatively speaking) thriving. Other leukodystrophies didn't match with his symptoms.

We wrote to specialists, saw neurologists at Children's Hospital, at Tufts, and at Mass General. One neurologist sent his MRIs to Holland, where the radiologist couldn't make a diagnosis but said that another family in the United States had a boy whose MRI appeared eerily similar. We contacted that family and found that the two boys shared many similarities, including that no one had any idea what their diagnosis was. Although this connection didn't move us any closer to a diagnosis or a treatment or cure, it still had enormous power. Finding this other family meant we weren't as overwhelmingly alone as we felt. We shared stories and had an immediate kinship, born out of our shared suffering in isolation. It was like finding a tiny, tiny burning ember in a very, very dark woods.

* * *

Ari died one day shy of what would have been his four-and-a-half-year-old birthday. Four and a half years would be a short life for any child—and for any parent—but because of his disabilities, Ari's capacities were far, far, far less than would have been normal for his age. So we lack more than most would after the death of a four-year-old. We don't have memories of conversations or understandings or verbal expressions of love. Ari never spoke; he could make sounds, but not words. Only Rob and I could understand the meaning of the few vocalizations he had—a sound to express want, a few numbers, a word for airplane—"nanna"—and a short exhalation that signaled "hi!"

Although I never was able to converse with him, Ari understood much more than he was able to express and did know how to communicate. He (and we) learned rudimentary American Sign Language. With this, he was able to express a few wants or needs: milk, cookie, and especially "more." This last sign was his favorite and captured his engagement and joy in the world. He signed "more" always, seeking more funny voices, more dancing, more music, more tickling, more giggling, just "more."

One day, Rob and I were driving home from a particularly devastating visit with some specialist. We had been told about Ari's neurologic findings and prognosis, neither of which was at all good. We were in the front seat talking about how scared we were of the future, unable to imagine how we'd go forward. "What are we going to do?" Rob asked aloud. His question was likely rhetorical, but I replied: "We're going to get up in the morning and pull on our shorts, and brush our teeth, and just keep going." And then I looked in the rearview mirror and there was Ari, smiling in his special way and signing "brush your teeth."

Ari turned four in September 2005. Compared to Jeremy he was doing well. He was thriving in our inclusive public preschool, was able to take a few steps with a walker and supervision, and was making progress learning signs. He could show that he understood how to count to ten, recognized shapes (including trapezoid and rhomboid, giving us a hint of his capacity) and colors, and letters. And he was a beautiful child, with a beaming smile and an easy, joyous disposition.

I remember that birthday in Kodachrome detail, likely because the pictures I took are saturated with the sunshine that fell on our deck in early September. And possibly because it was the last birthday he'd have, though I surely didn't know it then. Ari had woken from his nap in a cranky mood but emerged dramatically when he tore the wrapping paper off a present from our nanny and seemed to understand fully that it was a gift, and for him. Witnessing that moment of insight was sustaining; it felt like growth, which was joyous. It felt—just a little—the way a usual birthday party feels, like a marker of change and progress.

But Jeremy was not doing well. He wasn't growing. In fact, his pediatrician diagnosed him with "failure to thrive." At a year and a half, he weighed fifteen pounds, thirteen ounces, about as much as an average six-month-old. He'd gained nothing in the previous six months because he wasn't eating. Although he'd originally nursed and grown well, once weaned, he fought the bottle and the spoon. Feeding him was an exercise in misery. Rob and

I would sit in front of his highchair for two-hour stretches and feel as if we'd succeeded when we could coax two ounces of heavily fortified food to stay in. On top of all else we didn't have, we now were unable to feed our son. In fact, we were actively failing at it.

A dear friend had taught me what should be self-evident: food is love. In the context of caring for two disabled boys with special needs, the psychic toll of not being able to feed Jeremy was massive. Like all else, the painful, slow effort would have been difficult but endurable had it worked. But it never did. Hours of sitting and coaxing and cajoling led to no intake. I wept as I worked at it. The doctors recommended a feeding tube, but I resisted; we knew that there was nothing structurally wrong. Jeremy could eat and swallow. Although now, with the hindsight of how it eventually allowed him to live and thrive, the questions seem rhetorical to me, at the time they weren't: How could I put a feeding tube into a child who I knew had the capacity to eat? Why would I do this?

* * *

While this struggle was chronic and overwhelming, even its intensity was summarily eclipsed on March 11, 2006. Ari had been vomiting the day prior. And, although I can't fully remember it, something else must have been "off" because I decided to take him to the doctor. He was more lethargic, less engaged perhaps. I don't recall.

I remember sitting with him on my lap at the pediatrician's office. The pediatrician was concerned enough about the results of the fingerstick blood test that he sent us to the ER for hydration. After a few hours in the ER, a doctor came in and asked if my son had "finished his Popsicle." I recall being angered by this, that she didn't recall *my* child, because my son wasn't able to eat—anything, much less a Popsicle. I was alone, tired, and scared.

As I pushed Ari's stroller out of the ER after midnight, I passed the nurse who had done our triage. She'd been kind when we arrived—had made eye contact with Ari and now said something lighthearted about being glad we were going home. I recall wondering if I should share with her that Ari was still kicking his legs in a funny way. But I didn't stop. I also remember worrying if it was safe to walk to the garage a few blocks away. But there was no one at the security desk, and I wanted to get home, so I went out into the night on my own, pushing Ari's stroller down dark empty streets, a little scared. I wish now that the only darkness I would need to fear was that one.

At home, I put Ari on the soft carpet in the entry hall to remove his braces and sneakers before I carried him upstairs. He seemed not quite right to me, but, even then, that was a vague and ill-defined sense. It's only prescient in hindsight. Did he cry out in his sleep that night? Rob said he did. I slept late the next morning—it was a Saturday—and let Ari do the same. I stood in the kitchen with coffee and told Rob about all the parts of the ER visit that had been hard. At 9:30 we realized that it was unusually quiet, so we went upstairs. Ari was unresponsive in his crib. I called 911.

Although I knew that Ari was quite sick that morning, I was calm once we were at Children's Hospital. I thought "We made it. He's safe here. They'll figure it out." I even stepped out of his room to use the phone to call a friend. I hung up mid-sentence when I saw the crowd gathering around his bed: he was having seizures. The rest is a blur and plays in my head like a movie: Rob and I sitting on the side of the room, watching while a code was called, listening to the data being called out, knowing (as physicians ourselves) far too much about what the numbers meant. Did Rob say to me "he's dying"? I think so. I said "no, honey, no." It wasn't possible to believe such a thing. It was impossible. Rob knew it. I couldn't.

* * *

That night at home without Ari neither of us slept. We just clung to each other and cried. The world had been uncoupled from its axis; nothing made sense. The suddenness of Ari's death made it yet more incomprehensible. He'd been at school the day before, totally well. That fall—from health to death in less than twelve hours—was more than vertiginous. We'd fallen, too, into a dark space without meaning. In between reviewing and reviewing the previous days' events, trying to make sense of them, as if doing so would allow us somehow to rewrite history, I had moments of panic. "Where was Ari?" "Where had I left him, *alone*?" Even "knowing" that he was dead, I was distraught to think that he was alone in the funeral home. What kind of mother left her son in such a place alone? Ari wasn't, in fact, alone even there: because of Jewish tradition, we paid someone—a guardian—to sit with him. This still was not enough for me: I wondered aloud if we could go there. I was terrified to think of him there, scared, without his mother.

And I was cold; so very, very cold. I don't know words for the cold that took over my body after my firstborn son died. I'd say "chilled to my bones" but even that doesn't capture it. The cold was like a black hole in my body, the visceral inscription of my son's absence, the icy sensation of his death. No hug or blanket or cup of tea could touch it. I felt his loss in my body; I carried his absence with me.

We buried Ari two days later in an adult casket—the massive size of it made the unnatural timing of his death even more evident. Hundreds of people came to the funeral and to shiva. The house was teeming, filled simultaneously with both the noise of their words of consolation and the silence of the horror of it all. I found myself constantly introducing people to others, trying to answer unrelenting questions about why he died and how I was doing. I felt simultaneously numb and scared and overwhelmed and sad and angry. But mostly numb, I think. Or maybe that's how I felt after Jeremy died. I can't recall.

I do recall how much I came to hate the question, "How are you?" To say it rankled is to minimize its effect. Although I knew it was an expression of care, it felt like an assault, couched in terms that precluded my responding to its impact. How was I? I wanted to answer with expletives, with my own rhetorical question: "How the %^&# do you think I am?" A stickler for language, I found the mundanity of the question at best abrasive and, at worst, an existential question I was unable to answer. The *"how are yous?"* that populated our usual day-to-day world seemed foreign. I lived in another world, where a glib answer to that felt impossible. I didn't have language for my experience. That was part of "how" I was; I had no language.

I couldn't function after Ari's death. It's not that I couldn't do what is expected in a given day: I had to (Jeremy was alive then and needed a great deal of attention) and I did. I slept and ate and got things done (though I didn't return to my work for six months). I couldn't understand how the world still spun on its axis, how the sun still rose each day. The assumptions we make about our world eluded me. I didn't trust the floor to support me. I lived in dread that the ceiling would fall on my head, literally. The metaphorical nature of these fears didn't escape me, but neither did it diminish my terror. Nothing I'd relied on seemed reliable any longer. I hadn't lost faith in God, to the extent that I'd had such faith. Rather, I'd lost faith in the foundations that give our world stability and safety and predictability and form—the certainty that houses would stand, and gravity would work, and that four-year-old boys wouldn't die without warning.

I still don't fully remember the details of the weeks after Ari's death. I felt dislocated, as if I'd been suddenly transported to a place where the culture was foreign and unintelligible. I found it difficult to communicate with others—all, really, except for Rob—who lived in the "old" world. I didn't want to talk to anyone, in part because I didn't know how to. I made the mistake of picking up the phone one day and a work colleague—with good intentions, I'm sure—kept probing for what I was doing with my time: "Are you cleaning out his room?" "Are you going through his things?" Trying to respond to her reminded me of how I felt when I first moved to France as an exchange student: whatever sense I could make of things in my brain couldn't be translated to come out of my mouth, except this time my brain couldn't make any sense of things. I didn't answer the phone at all after that.

In the weeks and months after Ari died, Rob and I walked every day. Walking demanded nothing. We discovered private roads in our neighborhood and covered miles, plodding the same path day after day. We looked at the yards, the fences, the architecture. The familiar houses became words, and the streets sentences in the paragraph of our neighborhood, a physical space of familiar landmarks. Had there been soft earth, we would have carved our route in the ground, with its daily, predictable repetition. It was forward, in a way, but ultimately only circular; we kept going but never arrived anywhere but home. The walking became a daily routine, a familiar pattern, a repetition of steps; it was a ritual, translating into the physical a practice that was akin to prayer. It connected us to our world and each other without words or expectations. It was all we could do.

* * *

Life with "just Jeremy" was both heart-sickeningly easier than it had been previously and then tremendously difficult. Rob returned to work several months before I did, so I sat at home with my only disabled, nonverbal, tiny, failing-to-thrive son. The challenges of feeding him worsened, as did the pressure from his doctors to insert a feeding tube, along with the agony of considering a return to Children's Hospital and the idea of what felt like abandoning him to a team of doctors and the risks of general anesthesia. I didn't know what to do; I couldn't see any path to any kind of solution.

But Jeremy's "failure to thrive" was no euphemism; his fall off the growth curve was catastrophic—it was clear that he wouldn't live if we didn't intervene. So, at the end of May, two-plus months after we left Children's without Ari, we returned with Jeremy, and this time we walked out with our child after having a permanent feeding tube inserted in his stomach.

For the first few weeks, the feeding tube was a success, and I felt a modicum of hope. Jeremy started to gain weight at a clip, which was literally and visually sustaining. His tiny frame filled out, his face became fuller, highlighting his dimples, his skin a healthier, pinker hue. Although we still tried to encourage him to eat, the four-hour exercises in feeding failure were behind us. It was liberating. It didn't feel like a "new chapter," but it felt like we'd dodged a bullet. At least he was alive. "At least," as I said to Rob, "he won't die now."

But after the first few weeks, something changed, and Jeremy started to vomit with the infusions, which were supposed to happen four times a day. Something about the tube feeds was too much for him, and first once a day, and then twice, and then almost every time, he'd vomit during an infusion. Suddenly enteral nutrition became a bizarre game of strategy. If we let the infusion go on too long, he'd vomit it all up, and we'd lose any nutrition it provided. But if we stopped it early, we'd lose as well. He was still not getting enough calories. Rob and I devised ways to try to calculate how far we could go before we needed to call it quits. We thought Jeremy could sense the infusion, so we distracted him when we hooked it up; that only worked for a stretch. Then we decided that if he could hear the pump he was reminded, so we hid the tubing and pump and played music to drown out the sound. We played videos for him while the infusions went on. We played games. We sang. We danced. He vomited. I cried.

* * *

As the years passed after Ari's death, during the "just Jeremy" time, Rob and I began to talk about the future. Despite the challenges, or maybe because of them, we yearned for more—for another child, and for a sibling for Jeremy. Although it took years of intense and often difficult discussion, neither of us could close the book on the family we longed for. We weighed and measured every consideration and investigated every option to minimize the risks. Our decision might not have held up under rational scrutiny, but love isn't rational. Ultimately, despite all the reasons we "shouldn't have," our desire was strong enough to propel us forward, toward our third child.

Jonah was born on January 25, 2011, and, just like his two older brothers, he was a beautiful boy. But in contrast to them, he was healthy. I was astonished by how easy everything was. He slept, he nursed, he ate, he smiled, and giggled, and crawled and babbled, and he grew. Caring for him felt simple and straightforward. His body worked. Each scheduled visit to the pediatrician was normal, predictable, routine. And, although of course he still needed care at every stage, he soon became a buddy to Jeremy. Jonah never comprehended that his nonverbal, wheelchair-using brother wasn't "normal," so he treated him as he would have any brother; he tickled him and threw balls at him and gave him dive-bomb hugs. And Jeremy adored Jonah. He signed "baby" whenever Jonah came into the room and giggled at all the things he did, even when Jonah's skills quickly outpaced his.

So, our "Jeremy and Jonah family" took on a day-to-day structure. But especially as Jeremy grew, the physical components of his care became increasingly difficult. In addition to his feeding tube, he had four separate pairs of braces to keep his limbs functional—for feet, knees, and wrists. And he had to be placed into a "stander"—a contraption to keep him in an upright position for thirty minutes daily. The work to care for him grew harder and harder.

Jeremy graduated from using a stroller to a wheelchair at age six. The wheelchair offered many advantages and a slew of challenges. It had an attachable table (for school) and a backpack (for the feeding tube and supplies), and it could be folded. But it was also absurdly heavy and awkward. The safety mechanism that prevented Jeremy from tipping it backward also prevented me from lifting it up over a curb. Movement outside our house was simultaneously infinitely easier than it had been and also incredibly difficult. And that was when there was no snow on the ground.

* * *

The challenge of two sons with the same unnamed neurologic disorder who both die is that, despite their unique qualities, their lives and deaths blur and merge. It's hard to recall their particulars, which feels like yet another loss. And Jeremy's death was eerily similar to Ari's. It was December 24, and he had been vomiting. I am not sure what made me decide to call the doctor as vomiting wasn't unusual for him. Perhaps it was more intense or unrelenting. In part because of the looming holiday, the doctor recommended he come in. The pediatrician sent us to the ER, where fluids were given and a panel of blood tests were done. Jeremy perked up considerably, and the tests had normal results. Given our history, we were offered the option of staying overnight. But Rob and I both felt that Jeremy was better; he was giggling and interactive, and the tests were fine. So home we went.

The next morning was identical to the morning of Ari's death, though, of course, I did not know that then. When we went to get Jeremy, he was unresponsive. We called 911, and Rob went in the ambulance with him. After they left, I was strangely calm. I anticipated that he'd be kept overnight, so was packing things I'd need to stay there, when Rob called and said to hurry, that he was doing very poorly, being transferred to the ICU.

This is where the stories of Ari and Jeremy's deaths diverge. Ari died in the ER, not two hours after he arrived. Jeremy was transferred to the ICU immediately and died there some four or five hours later, after his status progressively worsened and after heroic measures failed to save him. I remember watching the team of doctors and nurses caring for him, sitting out of the way, listening. Sometimes they lowered their voices to discuss next steps or worries. I remember being annoyed that—as my son lay unconscious with a tube down his throat, IVs in his neck and leg, connected to monitors—the nurse breezily told us "He's doing great!" "Great," he wasn't doing, but I knew that my linguistic critique was irrelevant.

Jeremy's status deteriorated precipitously. In rapid succession, new, seemingly random issues arose: he was bleeding in his stomach; he had fluid around his heart; his lungs weren't working. They called out the results of a test to measure the amount of oxygen in his blood and it was dire. I remember dispassionately texting the numbers to a friend and a family member who were physicians. The numbers needed no narrative; they told the awful story.

The number of people in the ICU grew, as did the intensity of their efforts. At each awful juncture, the attending physician would come to sit with us, to review Jeremy's status. The penultimate time, he asked us if we wanted to consider ECMO—extracorporeal membrane oxygenation—a last ditch hope to "outsource" the work of the heart and lungs. The last visit was to say that there was nothing more that could be offered, there was no way to save Jeremy's life.

When Ari died, he was four years old, and the nurses helped put him in my arms so I could hold him. Although very small for his age, at nearly eleven years old, Jeremy was too large for this. The nurses removed all the tubes and monitors from his body, and Rob and I stood on either side of his bed, stroking his hair, kissing him, and trying to memorize his face.

There is no good way to say goodbye to one's dead child. This is what it is like: you cannot stay, and you cannot leave. Making the decision to leave the room feels like the worst form of abandonment. And yet, every moment you stroke your son's forehead, it becomes increasingly cool; the warmth that defines life diminishes. You do not want to remember your son cold and blue, so you force yourself to release your hand from his soft skin, knowing that you'll never be back.

The death of your second son takes you beyond the pale. The darkness and icy cold that I felt after Ari's death returned; sensations I now recognized. But that familiarity was another horror. All that is awful is compounded by the fact that you're accustomed with the plan this time. The calls to family and the rabbi and the funeral home are horribly routine. The death is incomprehensible, but the practical details are well-known. It even felt as if there wasn't space or room for comfort or condolence. Ari's death was so huge and overwhelming, it elicited a commensurate response. But Jeremy's? Another son dead? If the death of one son is enough to overwhelm people, the death of the second is silencing. There are no words.

Once again, during shiva, our house teemed with friends and family. It was horrendously similar to the days after Ari's death, but also different. Ari had been a preschooler when he died and had but a bare imprint outside of our home. But Jeremy was in fifth grade; he had a day-to-day world beyond us. Many of the mourners were from Jeremy's school: teachers and aides and parents, but also kids from his class, kids who—it turned out—were his friends. One after another, earnest, sweet fifth-graders came up to me and, through tears, told me how much they loved playing with Jeremy. Again, and again, I learned how sweet and funny they found him, how much they liked him—that they competed to see who his playground buddy could be each day. One girl told me that Jeremy was her "best friend." Age eleven, she told me that she planned to become a physical therapist because of Jeremy.

I had not realized, had not understood—frankly, had not had the capacity to imagine even—that Jeremy had friends. It shattered me to think that he'd had this community and that I hadn't known, that I'd been oblivious to this happy, "normal" part of his life. And, as much as I was devastated by this, by having to say to yet another parent and child, "I had no idea," I was also sustained: Jeremy had had more than I knew. He'd had fun at school, he'd been wanted there and knew it. He was loved by more than just his family. He'd had the joy of friendship and a richer life than I could conceive.

* * *

Bearing, loving, and losing Ari and Jeremy changed me. Raising two boys with profound disabilities and then burying them one by one has shifted my frame. Disability and death establish ease and health as extraordinary gifts. I know what matters, and I know what does not. I have little patience for the indiscriminate use of words that should be restricted. A dear friend taught me never to use the word "starving," as I am blessed never to be so, no matter how hungry I may feel. I think there are other words that should equally be reserved for times when they genuinely apply. I stiffen when I am told that the Little League Team loss is "tragic" or the cancellation of a much-anticipated event is "catastrophic."

Experiencing my life as charmed before my wedding meant that I relied on a set of assumptions or certainties. My losses cracked that open. The deaths of my sons shut me off from a worldview in which things work out in the end, and all is okay. I have learned how to navigate a world in which much of what I once construed as a "given," I no longer rely on. Death lurks everywhere. If my healthy ten-year-old sleeps late on a Sunday, I know that, along with the possibility that he's just tired and catching up on sleep, there is an equally likely possibility that he's died. I defer going upstairs because if it's the latter, I'd rather wait to find out.

I bristle when people suggest that I am a compassionate physician because of my losses. I find this reductive. It would be absurd if one could only be caring after profound suffering. But I understand the foundation of the question: from the crucible of my losses, have I not gained some pearl of insight that alters my care as a physician?

I think what I've gained is a ticket to an unseen world, a world in which many, many people—and many of my patients—live. When I care for patients, I am less focused on the medical narrative than I am on the human one. While of course I need to know the details of their medical concerns, my ear is tuned toward their suffering, their struggles, their isolation, their loss. Only a handful of the hundreds of patients for whom I care know my "story." Though I still struggle to answer my patients' routine questions about my family, I have learned to use the conditional tense, to be oblique, and—with as much breeziness as I can muster—to change the subject. But, even with those who know nothing, I have found that there is an invisible space in which we "see" each other. I ask questions differently than I once did. I pause more. And when I hear something—often quiet and small—that tells me that they, too, have visited a space of loss, I hold their gazes longer. Then we sit in silence, looking at each other, eyes often brimming, together.

I don't like reducing my experiences of loss to a set of lessons. I don't want to find any "silver linings." Finding the lesson in suffering seems at best to diminish the loss and, at worst, to make it somehow "worthwhile." There is nothing in what I went through and what I lost that was worthwhile. And so, even here with words, I struggle to make meaning from my experience. I struggle to make sense of it all. Michelangelo reportedly described his art as carving to find the sculpture hidden inside a block of marble. I have tried to carve from the marble of my life an understanding—a "piece"—that will somehow transcend the losses. But the marble refuses to budge, or perhaps it just crumbles; there is no sense to be made here, no neat resolution, no closure. Ari and Jeremy endure as absences. Their deaths don't give meaning to any narrative. They are just that—deaths: permanent, immutable, final. And so, I go forward carrying their absences, holding them with care, balancing cautiously as I step into my future.

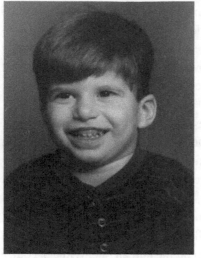

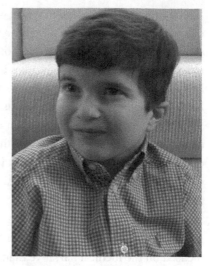

Ari, age 4   Jeremy, age 10

About the Author

Amy N. Ship, MD, MA, FACP, is a primary care doctor and Residency Program Director. Before attending medical school, Amy N. Ship studied English Literature at Swarthmore College and received a master's degree in art history from Columbia University. She trained in primary care internal medicine at Boston's Beth Israel Hospital and served as Chief Resident in that Program. Amy N. Ship worked at Beth Israel Deaconess Medical Center for more than twenty years, teaching medical students, residents, and faculty. In 2017, she became the Program Director for the Brigham & Women's Hospital Residency in Primary Care and Population Health co-sponsored by Atrius Health and the Department of Population Medicine at Harvard Medical School. She is currently the Director of Medical Education at Atrius Health, where she cares for patients in their Kenmore Internal Medicine practice. Amy N. Ship is Faculty Member of the Academy on Communication in Healthcare and serves as a Deputy Editor of the *Healing Arts* column at the *Journal of General Internal Medicine.* Amy N. Ship's teaching and writing focuses on humanism, communication skills, and physician well-being.

5

When the Loss Is Not Just Personal, but Is of One's Self

Julia H. Rowland

The soul always knows what to do to heal itself. The challenge is to silence the mind.

—Caroline Myss

Prologue

I am pausing here for a brief meditation on starting with a blank page which was never truly blank but simply hid the pain that was yet to be revealed. I have taken some deep breaths, as writing (and re-reading this narrative) leaves me breathless, whether from the sobs it induces or from holding my breath to see what is coming next, whatever I have dredged up and dragged myself back to, or, in the rush to put words on paper and capture conjured images, from literally forgetting to breathe.

I believe that (some, if not all) things happen for a reason, or at least the invitation to share my experience of loss and grief and healing. A larger force nudged the editors (Matt Loscalzo in particular) to reach out and me to say "yes."

It is now three years since the death of my son. Enough time to have distance and yet close enough to the pain and loss to still feel very raw. Enough time to realize that I need to take my mourning to a different level. To do that, I find myself wishing I had a tape recorder lodged in my head. I have had so very many conversations with myself since I was asked to contribute to this book. The hardest part is, of course, starting. When it comes to the causes and consequences of grief, there is no good place to begin. So, I am going to make a leap of faith and start telling the story.

Devastation

I am standing in my son's compact, spare, and surprisingly cold apartment; why is it so very cold in this room? The view from the eleventh story, which is stunning through big plate glass windows, looks south right down over Dupont Circle rooftops, toward the Washington monument. The structure would be illegal now when it comes to building heights in the District. Most shocking about this picture, I realize, are the sounds that surround me. I am swaying and loudly keening, and the cold I feel is part air conditioning, but largely the onset of shock. In the next room, the bedroom, lies the dead body of my beloved Boy-O.

How can I be here? How can this be happening? All I can think to say and utter is "No, no, no," as I rock myself back and forth, as though this mantra, this movement will magically bring him back. How can this possibly have happened? "No, no, no, no, no." Why did you do this Benji?! What were you thinking? How could you do this to me and your sister?!

You cannot be dead, and yet your body screams the reverse, the blood already pooling in dark reservoirs along your arms, your skin cold and clammy to the touch. Your face is set in a grimace, your expression makes me feel for a horrified and dizzying moment as though you perhaps have been murdered. Would this be better than the dawning realization that you have taken your own life? And yet there is no sign of struggle or chaos or disorder, except that the entire scene is so unreal, of a universe turned upside down. The violent personal struggle to stay alive, to stave off despair, to take control of your destiny is hidden from view.

I do not know from what unknown depth I draw the necessary composure to call my daughter to convey, with a barely contained and mounting sense of hysteria, the unimaginable. She is surprisingly calm at the other end (because, I learn later, she had feared the worst when I told her I was walking over to her brother's apartment). She is mobilizing already to pack up her Brooklyn-based family, husband and two small children, ages three and seven months, to come south to DC. The minute I hang up, I call her husband and leave an urgent message to please hurry home to care for her, her brother has died. The minute she hangs up, she turns around and calls my best friend in DC to please go be with me in this grim apartment and help take me home. There is a fleeting moment when I acknowledge and give silent thanks for the fact that neither my mother nor my husband, Ben's grandmother and father, are alive and will not have to face the violent trauma that has taken place. I barely have a grip on my own grief; I am not sure I could have sustained theirs for their adored grandchild and child. Summoning 911 comes next for me.

Then there are the police and rescue team. They push me aside and invade Ben's bedroom but realize quickly that we are all hours too late (six or seven at least, the coroner would ultimately pronounce). Then they are busily hunting for a suicide note and scanning for drugs or prescription medication bottles (of which it turns out there are many). There is no note, no reason, no voice from beyond the dead, but they keep circling back to the handwritten message I left Ben on his living room table letting him know how proud I was of him for hanging in for the full month-long detox program for which he had enrolled and how deeply I loved him, and, oh yes, that I had left provisions for him in the fridge, raw vegetables with and ready for dipping, fruit, cold cuts and multigrain bread, milk, the makings of a simple meal and snacks. There is no suicide note. No explanation of what he was thinking and feeling, why he has left us. He is simply and utterly and irretrievably gone. Did he mean for, know this would happen? Is this just a terrible mistake? Was he confused and accidentally overmedicated himself? Indeed, the medical examiner's initial summary would read quetiapine (the generic name for Seroquel, an antipsychotic) and diphenhydramine (the over-the-counter cold medication, e.g., Benadryl) intoxication as the immediate cause of death.

This is the scenario—and repetitive soundtrack—that will play, like a movie on a looping reel, for months to come, at the drop of a hat, and even today at unexpected moments. I see this happening in slow motion and me in it, like a spectator at times or at others physically present again, overcome with grief and loss, doubling over with physical and emotional pain. I want to stop the movie and roll back the tape. Can't we have a different ending to this? Surely there could be a different ending.

The first hours, days, and weeks after Ben's death are a blur. I remember the early days of this period feeling as though I was drowning in a sea of grief. I would struggle up a wave only to realize the horizon was limitless and find myself thrown back down into a trough of sorrow. My cherished friend Ellie shows up at Ben's apartment to gently spirit me away from this place of horror. I am devastated that she has to be there, that I am there, as they carry Ben's body out in a blue body bag to the morgue. It is all I can do to keep from grabbing, holding on tight, and traveling along with him. I cannot remember how I drove home? Once home, there is the constant flow of friends and neighbors and colleagues who come to share the grief, mourn, comfort as best they can. Then Katie arrives with her family, and we clutch one another as though our lives depended on this hanging on.

Her amazing, beautiful, smart, and accomplished tribe of women, friends since her undergraduate days at Columbia University, begin to arrive to nurse and nourish and provide a buffer for us from immediate reality. The flow of what I have come to call the "administrivia" of death is stunning: picking up Ben's personal effects from the city's bleak morgue, identifying his body at the funeral home prior to cremation (I freak out that he may appear as he did when I found him, but underestimate the skill of the undertakers that enables them to bring calm and order to his red-bearded good looks), ordering death certificates, launching the endless notifications of his passing, arranging for a memorial service, getting through the memorial service where so many loving friends showed up (oh, dearest Ben, did you know how beloved you were to so many?), packing up his small apartment—that pitiless still life that was his refuge with its meagre, largely second-hand, tangible testaments to a foreshortened life—and shutting the door to the empty space behind me. I literally rock myself to sleep at night in tears that only that back-and-forth motion can begin to soothe. I fret over where he is, might have gone?

I worry that his being, essence, soul if you will, is unsettled and that, while untethered from our sentient world, cannot leave us. The worry unnerves me, irrational as I know it to be. Katie and I both sense Ben is about during those early days and fully expect to see him in dreams or some type of manifestation. Where can he have gone? Is he as shocked to be there as we are not to have him among us? Is he going to be taken care of wherever it is he has gone?

Though raised in the church (Presbyterian), I do not consider myself deeply religious but rather profoundly spiritual, anchored by a steadfast belief in our respective humanity, kindness, and oneness, our deep connection to each other and nature. I am nonetheless comforted by the young minister, Chris, from the Georgetown Presbyterian Church, who will lead the service for Ben. In many ways, he is just like Ben: tall and lanky, a bike rider and rock-music lover, broad smiling, good humored, also thirty-three, and a dedicated outreach worker.

In college, in Portland, Oregon, Ben started volunteering to join peers who walked the streets in pairs on set evenings to provide outreach to lost young people. For his senior thesis, he would research and write about the loss of access to healthcare services that would impact sex workers when business was conducted via the internet versus the sidewalk. His people skills led him later to become an assistant teacher in classrooms designed for behaviorally challenged children in the public middle school system, those who could not be mainstreamed. At the end of his life (a hard phrase even to type), he served as an outreach staffer for a DC-based organization, Pathways to Housing, that helped homeless people make their way through the system to more permanent housing options. His gift was making people feel they were important. There was no judgment or condescension in his exchanges: he was simply there to help. He was duly proud of his work and the successes achieved in securing safe homes for a handful of individuals. Since the onset of the pandemic, I have thought often about how distressed Ben would have been for the well-being of his clients and been grateful that he was spared this nightmare. Both the risk of virus exposure due to his work and the imposed isolation due to the virus would have been devastating to him. Looking back, I have found myself wishing that Chris, our pastor, and Ben would have made a connection after my husband's death, when we first met Chris. Perhaps Chris could have helped Ben. Perhaps, perhaps . . . such wishful, wistful thoughts.

The question of where Ben is haunted me from the start and abides with me. I remain worried he is "caught" in some limbo universe because of the psychic violence with which he left. Chris is reassuring. But what helps most is talking months later and again a year later with a Shaman that Katie was working with spiritually and also as an editor for her book on her Shamanic tradecraft. Kerry, a skilled and deeply experienced pathfinder who both sees and senses Ben, tells me that he is fine, that he wants me to know this, and that he has work to do in his other life. Importantly, he is not stuck or lost but at peace and happy. I ignore the rational voice in my head that wants to reason away this reassurance as "magical thinking" and embrace the empathic and deeply sensed feeling that this interpretation is correct. Kerry also encourages me to listen to some Gregorian chants; she is not sure why, but they provide relief and comfort as they wash over me, a reminder to myself that music has always fed me and spoken to my heart and soul. There is a reason why I went to Oberlin, a college with a Conservatory.

Grieving

Right from the start and in the lasting wake of this inconceivable loss, the unrelenting cascade of "what if's" and "if only's" come pouring in. I can only liken this to falling down a rabbit hole, an experience shared by many

facing loss—especially when this is to suicide, I later discover. I find myself reflexively labeling these thoughts as I have been taught as intrusive
thinking; a common response to trauma. While they are indeed invasive, for
me, the questions are also part of my desperate search to make sense of what
happened, find something or someone to blame (often me), find some rational explanation for what was a profoundly irrational event/act. What if
I had insisted that he stay with me when he was discharged two weeks earlier from his treatment program? What if I had only called him earlier in the
week to check in? What if I did not take no for an answer when I invited him
for dinner on Sunday and he declined? Why didn't he call me to let me know
he felt so terribly sad and despairing? If only we had been able to get him in
to see a better therapist? If only he had been willing to try lithium? If only
he had gone to a treatment center where they treated those with a dual diagnosis? This is how I could rewrite the script. But how far back would I need to
go to stop the excruciating ending? Likely in utero, the quietly rationale voice
of the developmental or, as affectionately referred to, "womb-to-tomb" psychologist in me would reason.

Ben, who shared his given name with his father and an uncle, was the
sweetest and most cheerful of babies. A December baby by birth (Sagittarius),
he was also the quietest of infants. So quiet, indeed, that once when I was
out walking with him in his perambulator, a next-door neighbor, whose four
girls I had grown up babysitting, leaned over his carriage and wondered was
he always so quiet? My answer was an unhesitating yes. "Oh," my neighbor
remarked, "you will find out how quiet he is when you have to ask him to
move out when he's thirty-five." What a strange reflection, an exchange that
was seared in my memory: Was it some curse? As it happens, my own father
was thirty-six and still living at home when he met and married my mother,
sixteen years his junior!

Towheaded and bright, with a doting sister four years his senior, and
adoring and accomplished parents, young Ben's life seemed charmed, comfortable in every way. He was one of those rare boys who had the ability to
travel comfortably with the jocks and the nerds without prejudice from either. He was also a champion for the underdog, whoever that might be in
any given moment. In looking back, which I—and, it turns, out most suicide
survivors do endlessly (obsessively) in the wake of this type of trauma—I
tried to figure out when things began to go wrong. Ben's sister, in processing
her own grief, wrote beautifully about this in her piece for *Guernica* entitled,
"Where Disease Stopped, and My Brother Began" (June 21, 2019).

Yes, he seemed sad in junior high and we found him a counselor whom he grudgingly saw briefly until both decided there was nothing to work on (or possibly with?). Changing schools for high school was the right decision, as was his pursuit of plans to go to Reed College, out in Oregon. He grew to love the Pacific Northwest. But it was also out there, after college, that cracks in what was an otherwise happy existence began to show. He experienced a devastating breakup of a relationship in which he was deeply committed, yet came home minimizing this and with ideas for coming back east to help out with the care of his father (which he would eventually do in 2013, moving from Portland to DC) who at that point himself was not doing well mentally or physically. He also started drinking too much.

Upon reflection, this classic manic-depressive pattern started slowly but would become more intense in the decade to follow, with the highs—that ranged from grand plans for new programs he would lead at his former high school to engage students more meaningfully in social service programs, to holding a pop-up music event to raise money to teach the homeless in DC to repair bicycles and enable them to become independent physically and financially, to housing all of DC's homeless in the Trump International Hotel (conceived as a grand political gesture)—becoming higher and accompanied by uncontrolled bouts of drinking and the lows becoming more fathomless and difficult from which to recover.

He tore through two more intense relationships, the final one ending in a proposal of marriage, days after which he went missing. We eventually found him (a useful albeit unnerving benefit of the internet and its tracking ability), and I pretty much dragged him to what would be his first of two voluntary in-patient hospitalizations. It was devastating on so many levels. It hit me with profound sorrow and disbelief as I drove home from the hospital that I had participated in the psychiatric admission of all three members of my immediate family: my daughter in the fall of 2000, in the wake of a deep depression and suicidal thoughts secondary to a vicious sexual assault; my husband in 2008, after a late-life psychotic break; and now my son, in November 2017. I felt profoundly helpless as a mother and wife and as a psychotherapist. Psychology was my chosen field, and yet my training was of little use in warding off the disastrous events that affected each of my immediate family members in turn, daughter, husband, and son. I felt acutely responsible each time for getting it right; specifically, for finding the best care and ensuring good outcomes. That said, my understanding of the dynamic behind these episodes and my appreciation for how little we truly understand about mental illness, has likely helped me be more compassionate with myself in hindsight.

The pain at Benji's admission to care was compounded as this came days before I was due to go up to New York City to be with my daughter, his sister, for the arrival of her second child. Having to choose between the profound and competing needs of my two children tore me apart. Because Ben was hospitalized and thus "safe," I headed north for Brooklyn. It was only after the baby was born, beautiful Alma St. Joan (little soul savior literally!) that the real dilemma hit: Should I stay in Brooklyn as I had promised Katie to help out with her little family for a couple of weeks as she recovered from the caesarian section, or return to DC to provide a safe harbor to and over-sight of Ben? I felt like Meryl Streep in *Sophie's Choice*. I ended up staying in Brooklyn and recruited one of Ben's friends to stay with him at my house until I came back to DC. It was a lame solution as his friend bailed early, probably under pressure from Ben that he was "fine," and Ben ended up back in his apartment alone. I was not a happy camper about the entire sequence of events. I was, in fact, totally stressed out about wanting to pick up and fly home to care for Ben and anguished about not being fully "present" fol-lowing the joyous arrival of my second grandchild, Alma, and the tender care needed by Katie and her family, including my first grandchild, Finn, aged two and a half.

Christmas, a season that brings both my children's birthdays, was deeply fraught that year (2017). Ben, more or less back on his feet, and I both went up to Brooklyn, but he said he was staying with friends. He would arrive at Katie's Brooklyn house staggering drunk early Christmas morning. I took him in; how could I not? I was terrified of what would happen to him in the streets. But Katie and her husband Eddie were enraged. Mad that he could be so disruptive of their lives, scared silly underneath of what was happening to him. And so it went, steadily downhill.

In March, Ben was put on probation at his job for missing work. In April, he was back in the hospital for depression. In May, he finally agreed to enter a residential program, but the one he chose within his insurance policy, while well-reputed, was primarily for those with drug and alcohol abuse problems. Ben's problem was not that he did not abuse alcohol: he did. It was that he used it to self-medicate when he was manic. The rest of the year, the other five or so months, he was stone cold sober. Did they realize this at the center? I will never really know. A knowledge gap that still haunts me. He stuck it out regardless. He wanted so to be and feel better. It makes me weep to this day to think how very hard he was working to be well.

Recovery and Healing

The death of a child, by whatever means, is to me the most traumatic of losses, something I witnessed and came to believe when I began my oncology career working in the Pediatrics Department at Memorial Sloan Kettering Cancer Center. Child-loss flies in the face of our steadfast belief that our children and grandchildren are supposed to bury us, their parents and elders, and not the reverse.

How do I, will I, am I going to live with this loss? There are days now three years later that I am not sure how I am still here. The why is easier and, at a deep level, is what anchors me in this world. My daughter and her three little ones. They are my heart. At a minimum, I could never do to Katie what her brother, not by choice, did to us: left us so grievously mourning.

What was helpful about Ben's treatment program was the weekend they held for family. Here I not only had a chance to tell Ben how very much I loved him and admired how hard he was working on recovery, including consistent, coin-earning attendance at his AA program, but also to know the love was mutual. While I had known from my own training the challenge of addiction, I also learned first-hand, listening to the patients and families share their experiences, that addiction truly was a hijacking of the amygdala, a case of the brain on fire.

Beyond some reading as part of my training as a psychologist, I really did not understand the underpinnings of bipolar disorder. Although, curiously, I had encountered it before, something I would only remember after Ben's death. The woman who introduced my husband and me to one another developed the illness a couple of years after we married. I was among the first to notice that she seemed to be becoming strange or, as I would realize later, manic. Her friends, including my husband, all just said, "Oh that's just Jane (not her real name) being Jane." I finally blew the whistle and called her brother who was a physician, sharing details of what I thought was very alarming and potentially self-harmful behavior. He came and took her back home to the Midwest where she was successfully treated, going on to marry, adopt a daughter, and lead a full life on medication.

It was only in the wake of Ben's suicide that I threw myself into the literature about the disease, dragging my way through Kay Jamieson's book, *An Unquiet Mind*, dissecting her own struggle with the illness. And also, the autobiography of Hope Jahren, *Lab Girl*, that chronicles her effort to create and advance a career as a female scientist, a geobiologist, and, more specifically, a paleobotanist at that, while trying to manage her often out-of-control bipolar disorder. Surprisingly, if you Google "Hope Jahren," there is little mention of her mental health despite this being a critical and candidly shared aspect of her part-science, part-memoir volume, both of which—the science and her life—are fascinating and beautifully recounted (see https://www.youtube.com/watch?v=UJa8dzBAhmY). But both Kay and Hope survive. Therein lies the rub for me.

Reading has helped, at least the left-brain side of me, my efforts to understand if not adapt to (accept?) the terrible effects of this disease. Perhaps it assuages slightly—if not entirely effectively—the guilt about not being able to save Ben from himself. As an oncology professional, my reading made me realize that we know far more about cancer and how the disease and its treatments affect the mind and body than we do mental illness. That makes me angry. Would we be kinder to those who thought about and attempted suicide but survived if we realized that suicide is akin to a heart attack of the brain, as I have heard it described? Compassion is needed not just for self, but also for the loved ones we lose to mental illness.

Ben came by his illness naturally. He was part of a line of men on his father's side of the family with psychiatric histories. His grandfather and father both were hospitalized for psychiatric care. So, too, briefly was his uncle, his father's younger brother who, although never fully diagnosed, has struggled a lifetime with mental health issues and a rocky, at times tempestuous and contentious, relationship with family. Maybe this is really where it all began? The deck was stacked against him. This thought is small comfort. Given this genetic loading, I keep thinking how difficult it might have been for Ben to feel he could not overcome his illness, that he could pass on this scourge if he had children.

Numb in the weeks after his death, I finally decide to go see a therapist. I am lucky and find someone who is a good match for me. And yet, the process is so very difficult and painful. That forty-five minutes a week is the only time I talk about Ben's death. It is like a small escape valve where the pressure is released and the tears allowed to flow. It is emotionally draining and frequently physically uncomfortable at times; my gut gnarled up and my sides aching. It is months before I can go to a session and not instantly dissolve into a puddle of tears and outright sobbing. I feel as though I should come with my own box of tissues.

I am not an easy patient, and I do not feel at ease being a patient. As a mental health professional myself, I struggle with the need to protect my therapist from my overwhelming sorrow. It is hard for me to *be* a patient. It is not that I fear being vulnerable. Rather, I want to be a good patient (for her, not me) and fret that she may feel bad about herself because she cannot assuage my grief. I am inconsolable; how do you treat that? I worry that I will drown her in my sorrow. I realize as I write this that, yes, it is funny I should feel this way. As a psycho-oncologist, my own clients are exclusively cancer patients/survivors or their loved ones, commonly dealing with the existential issues of premature death and loss imposed by a cancer diagnosis and its treatments. Yet I do not feel overwhelmed by their grief and loss; rather I am moved to compassion, feel privileged to bear witness to their struggle, and know (now even more deeply than before) that just being able to sit and listen is healing.

It takes me a year of solo therapy to even consider a grief group for those who have lost a loved one to suicide. I have to smile as this is so very ironic. As a support group leader in my current work, I know first-hand the rich and healing value of groups and even tout their benefits to prospective members, though also cautioning that they are not for everyone. Part of the uniquely therapeutic effect of these groups is the sense of suffering on the same plane as other members. I dragged my heels about signing on, knowing I would again find it hard to step out of my professional self to be a group member. And it remains hard to rein in my professional self. Harder still, however, is hearing in detail how many ways there are for people to take their own lives. There is a perverse sort of downward comparison that can occur, where there is a moment when you think, oh thank God my loved one did not hang or shoot herself in front of me or throw himself off a bridge. Listening to others' stories is a form of retraumatization. At the same time, there is deep community in the experience of a loss that others find so very difficult to hear: suicide. What can you say to someone who has lost a loved one to suicide? My wise group taught me one special phrase of kindness that has stayed with me: "I am so sorry (insert here the name or relation to the person lost) was in such pain."

Aside from the deep kindness and profoundly shared injury and loss, the group has also helped me tame the impulse to blame myself for Ben's death, helped heal my sense of guilt, reminded me to have self-compassion. I think that for mental health professionals, many—myself included—are particularly burdened by the belief that we could and should have been able to save our loved one. Among our shared stories in group, so much was done to help our loved ones: counseling and medications and understanding and hospitalization and support and understanding. And still these deaths occurred. Ben's death on June 14, 2018, occurred not long after the suicides of Kate Spade and Anthony Bourdain. I remember thinking that here were two amazingly accomplished individuals with (presumably) full and rich lives (at least from the public perspective) and likely (assumed again) full access to all the best possible care needed, and yet this did not protect them from personal pain. The fact that Ben lived to be thirty-three, as my grief group members whose loved ones died at a much younger age have reflected for me, may be remarkable given how challenging his illness was and says much about the love and care he received. I am humbled by and grateful for their healing words.

I still struggle with the language of loss. The label "suicide" connotes a sense of responsibility, as though the person had a choice, was cogent at the time of the act or even rational. Technically, Ben died of Seroquel toxicity, the drug he was prescribed and taking for his illness. There was no note, there was not proof of intentionality; it was a drug overdose. I railed for a while about this, not that the outcome would be any different. He had died, unwittingly or not, at his own hands. Suicide is viewed as a crime, a bizarre one where the victim is also the perpetrator. Life insurance companies consider it grounds for denying coverage. And, in truth, we will never know the truth. It does not alter the anguish of knowing he was in such pain and that he felt helpless in the face of this. Believing that downing a lot of pills was a last act of control is but small comfort for the gaping hole of his absence.

I Am No Stranger to Loss

My seminal and unwelcome introduction to losing a loved one was the untimely death of my father when I was eighteen. He had his third massive coronary two months after he retired and just weeks before he and my mother were to set off around the world to adventure. Aside from being profoundly shocked by his death, I learned the cruel fact that life inexorably goes on even when you think the world should have come to an absolute standstill at so momentous an event. I still miss my father and, at every major, especially joyous life event (college graduation, marriage, births of his grandchildren, receiving awards, etc.), wonder what he would have thought or said. I know he would have been proud as I was graced to be on the receiving end of his unconditional love. I remember him walking by my room at home, peering in and pointing at me saying I was such a hardworking student, when in fact hearing him, I had just tucked out of sight the junk romance novel in which I was enthralled and picked up a nearby textbook. I picture him at my graduation from high school, his Olympic-level water polo player's barrel chest puffed out proud, photographed next to me holding my diploma.

This early trauma was followed in my young adult years by the loss of cherished friends: my first serious adult boyfriend, lost first to his realization that he was gay and then fully when he succumbed in the early years of the epidemic to AIDS; our fun and delightfully dilettantish next door neighbor who died suddenly of a blood clot post-surgery; and my good buddy from graduate school whose statistical wizardry helped me successfully analyze the data for my doctoral thesis and co-author with me of an award-winning paper of the findings, but whose sedentary, high-fat, chain-smoking lifestyle took him out prematurely of irreversible heart disease. I still grieve for each of these gentle souls.

Leading up to young Ben's death, in sad sequence, were the death of my mother and husband. My mother died in September 2014, at the fine, well-traveled age of ninety-three, but following seven horrible years of impaired and increasingly dependent living resulting first from a devastating stroke and, at the end, from a catastrophic fall that left her quite literally in pieces. It was a terrible way to go and most cruel in the end. My brilliant, multilingual, life-long learner of a mother became trapped in a body that slowly betrayed her and then refused to let her die. My husband, Ben's father, also Ben, died the beginning of March 2016, after a two-year, all-hands-on-deck battle with metastatic colorectal cancer. My mother's passing was a deep release for all. By contrast, my husband's death was a painful and, at the end, shockingly swift process that left us all reeling. For Benji in particular, though he understood there was no cure in sight and his father was suffering, letting his father go took every ounce of courage he could muster. At some level, I think he believed he could save his father, and, when he could not, the affront to his ego was not trivial. In the case of my father's death, and that of my mother by whose side I stayed as she made her passage out of this realm, and, minutes after the fact, my husband's death, I had witnessed the dying process and seen what death looked like. That was part of the horror of going into young Ben's bedroom: the moment I touched him, I knew right away he was dead. The only grace to be clawed from these two preceding deaths is that they ended the deep suffering of my mother and husband, and neither lived to experience the tragedy of young Ben's suicide. I take small blessings where I can.

We have language for many losses and "new" statuses. In a three-year span, I was orphaned, widowed, and then retired. I stepped down from my eighteen years in the federal government at the end of September 2017, just as things were beginning to be truly crazy for Ben. In anticipation of this big change, I panicked at the thought of retiring, so instead of taking time off— yes, surely earned after all the years working in the field—I leapt back into another job, walking out of the National Cancer Institute offices on a Friday afternoon and showing up the following Monday morning at Smith Center for Healing and the Arts. What was I thinking? The answer is, I wasn't: I was panicking about who I would be without work to define me. In my right mind (and my hard-won wise advice for anyone considering the same), I should have taken three months off to think about what I really wanted to be doing and laze about the beaches of Bali.

Benji's death only served to untether me further and was compounded— as I look back now—by the big losses leading up to it. Who was I if not the parent of two children? Even now, I can be momentarily tongue-tied when people I do not know well ask me if I have any children. I cannot answer them without mentioning Ben, and yet the pain on both sides is always visible: it is hard for me to say and hard for others, strangers, to hear.

Beyond knowledge and familiarity with death, a strong buffer to the pain has been family.

Pulling, at times dragging me through the motions of "normal" life has been the magnet of my grandchildren. It is their unbounding joy, laughter, wonder, and curiosity, ever-changing little beings with the ability to live fully in the present that has been my core, my sense of purpose, what keeps me here, wanting to be here with and among and for them, along with the knowledge that I could never wittingly do to my daughter Katie, what Ben unwittingly (and I will always believe *unwillingly*) did to us: leave us abandoned and bereft with no real explanation, not that I am sure any explanations are soothing.

A further source of solace is my work. Yet it is also my hurdle to fully grieving. I returned to work six weeks after Ben died. The structure helped, as did keeping busy, and my cherished colleagues were gentle and caring.

Still, driving by Ben's apartment (which I quickly realized I did daily once I returned to work, and quickly sought new pathways to the office) and walking in what I considered his neighborhood were regular prompts to grief.

Why is it that caregivers have such trouble caring for themselves? This is a common topic in the cancer caregiver support group I am privileged to facilitate, and it seems to be a theme with healthcare providers in particular. We are great at giving advice: "You need to take care of *you* first. Put your oxygen mask on before you reach to help others with theirs." But many of us are really deficient at taking it. At least that is true for this healthcare provider!

A final source of comfort and healing has been the remarkable set of friends and colleagues who have seemingly appeared (although they were probably there all along) in the wake of Ben's death. Small acts of kindness— the random note to let me know I am thought of sent months after Ben's death, the favorite baked recipe arriving freshly cooked at the front door, the invitation just to come out and walk—each have a profound impact. Being willing to be with me when I am racked by grief—and *not* telling me everything will be all right—is a sacred act.

Unfinished Business

Ben's battered yet sleek Gitano racing bike still sits in my book-lined study, though I have removed his size eleven shoes from my front hall and put them up on a high shelf in the closet. I have yet to tackle the boxes he had stored in my attic, which include his box of eight-track equipment, playing card collections, electronics, and miscellaneous files. And there are days when I need to hear his voice once more and will call his phone number (which I still pay for) just to hear him tell me to leave a message and that he will get back to me. He never does. But I will sometimes also listen to my own messages left for him. I know that Katie frets that the killer genes in our family may have made their way into the pool that produced her three beautiful offspring. I, in turn, live with (and likely always will) worry about her health and sanity, especially in a world of pandemic chaos with little ones, a husband, and big career to manage. We dance around our concerns for one another, not wanting to burden or frighten one another with the depth of our sorrow, occasionally revealing that we still struggle privately with the loss of our Boy-O. I believe that time helps, but it is not a cure; there is not a cure for loss and grief. Rather, we find new ways to abide reality, accommodations that age and shift as we do, even though Ben will forever be thirty-three, a fact that is also hard to get around.

Epilogue

Letting the genie out of the bottle is always easier than putting it back in. Like the Ancient Mariner, I have told my tale and now, hopefully, can move on for a time without the urgent need to recount this story afresh. Loss lives in me that way; tucked away neatly in a corner of my mind and heart until summoned. I am not always sure what will provoke the images or waves of sadness that lap at me when my mind drifts to thoughts of my son. Part of me hopes that this will always be true as it is a way to hold on to this soul so dear to me until we are reunited in some other universe or dimension. Meanwhile, he shows up in subtle ways, in the coin I find on the sidewalk, the sense that I have left my glasses on a closet shelf (who could possibly remember that!?), the urge to pull out a dollar when I encounter a homeless person or a musician busking in the subway.

No doubt this volume will demonstrate to its readers that there is no one way to live with, through, and beyond loss and grief. We each find our own path, trying, as we are wired to do, to make sense of the tragedy and striving to find continued meaning, purpose, and love without the presence of that particular significant other or others, or piece of ourselves, or belief. The essence of this work is finding a narrative you can live with, a means to survive survivorship as it were. Having much adored grandchildren, a part-time job and work that I love, good and enduring friends, and, for me, the realization that I have in my life to find ways to honor my son's passion, compassion, and caring, all keep me going, racing ahead often, hurtling myself into the days, but at times, grateful just to be able to put one foot in front of the other until the tears stop and the loss settles. I hope dear reader, this is or will be true for you as well.

> For it's our grief that gives us our gratitude
> Shows us how to find hope, if we ever lose it.
> So ensure that this ache wasn't endured in vain: Do not ignore the pain.
> Give it purpose.
> Use it.
> —Amanda Gorman, US Poet Laureate (*The Miracle of Morning*)

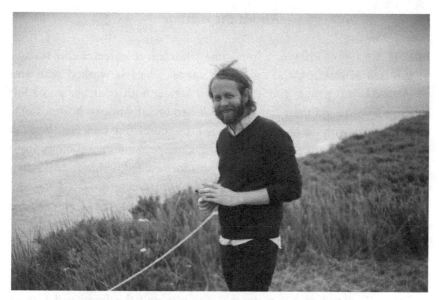

Ben, my beloved Boy-O, Summer 2017

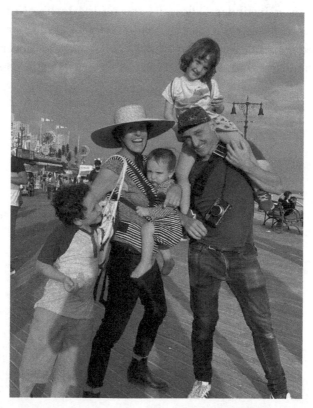

Katie and family, Coney Island, NY, October 2021. My 'why'

About the Author

Julia H. Rowland, PhD, is a long-time clinician, researcher, and teacher in the area of psychosocial aspects of cancer. She has worked with and conducted competitively funded research among both pediatric and adult cancer survivors and their families, published broadly in psycho-oncology, and co-edited, with Jimmie Holland, the groundbreaking text, *Handbook of Psychooncology*. She received her PhD in developmental psychology from Columbia University and completed a postdoctoral fellowship in psychosocial oncology at Memorial Sloan-Kettering Cancer Center (MSKCC), where she went on to hold joint appointments in pediatrics and neurology. Across her career, she was privileged to champion a number of firsts. She helped develop and was the first Director of MSKCC's Post-Treatment Resource Program, an innovative, nonmedical resource for patients and their families beyond active treatment. She was the founding Director of the Psycho-Oncology Program at Georgetown University and the Lombardi Cancer Center in Washington, DC. She was also the first full-time Director of the National Cancer Institute's Office of Cancer Survivorship. Currently, she serves as Senior Strategic Advisor to Smith Center for Healing and the Arts, a DC–based nonprofit that provides integrative services to cancer survivors and their families and advocates for evidence-based care in the community.

6

Speechless

Matthew Loscalzo

In June 1973, at the age of forty-nine, my mother, Concetta Greco Loscalzo, died a miserable, painful death. There were no angels or devils in this story, but there was a conspiracy of silence, and I was an active accomplice.

From the start, losses have made me who I am. The drive and agony of writing these memory-stories remain as hard to write as not. At this point in my life, there is no choice. I have no children of my own to carry these genes or the stories forward. The agitated voices within me will not stay silent.

Here are the scenes, never so openly shared with anyone (including me).

Big John

It was a typically sticky, hot, and bright Bronx summer in 1960. The borough was filled with Eastern Europeans, Irish, Italians, Puerto Ricans, and increasing numbers of African Americans escaping from the putative genteel South. The Clason Point Housing Projects were fairly new, and most of the inhabitants, including my family, felt lucky to be there, especially after departing from the tired, dilapidated, walkup tenements deteriorating by the moment.

I was eight years old and on my way to work. My boss was named John. Except no one called John, John. He was "BigJohn," like it was all one word. Big John was both big and tall, and I was small, not only because I was eight, but because I *am* small. Big John smelled like he'd fallen into a bottle of cheap men's cologne. He ran a vegetable market—a space too raw to be called a store. Everyone talked loudly, mostly in numbers, lots of numbers. As a New Yorker, I was amazed by the exotic diversity of summer fruits and vegetables. I preferred the seasonal summer fruits, especially the fuzzy peaches. Figs and I were already well acquainted because, in the neighborhood, people who lived in private homes often grew figs. During the summer, these trees had broad, flat, outstretched, three-fingered leaves. Come winter, they were lovingly wrapped in blankets of thick black industrial plastic, laid to rest before resurrecting in spring. Big John let me weigh the fruits and vegetables, but only at his direction. I could never quite figure out which numbers meant pack the fruits and vegetables and which he would simply write down on small pieces of paper. After a few weeks of "working," Big John started telling people, "Have you met my son, Matty? He is going to be a lawyer." No one bought it, as we looked nothing alike, but it meant a lot to me, that he would be proud to call me his son. At the end of each day, however long I was there, twenty minutes or a few hours, Big John would give me a bunch of quarters from the big black steel register. The silver was shiny and heavy in my pocket. I was rich!

But there were limits to my relationship with Big John. I remember where I was standing when I told Big John, "I want to be just like you." And I did. Surprisingly, this did not go over well, at all. His uncharacteristic response was immediate, with all the due consideration of any primitive reflex of a Bronx bookie: "You are going to college and you will be a lawyer." This was the best time in my eight-year-old life. Hard work, counting lemons, weighing potatoes—this was a part of my life that was now even more deeply engrained. My father worked two full-time jobs. Most of my relatives worked more than one job. Now, I was working, too. We were all connected. My emerging self-concept—smart, assertive, hard worker—connected me to the powerful people bigger than myself.

One Saturday in September, as excited as ever, I rushed to Big John's and arrived right on time at 8:00 A.M. I found the gates cold and locked tight. The market was empty. Where did everything go? No Big John, no vegetables, no customers. Only this core of empty confusion and searing nausea. The deep connection of the previous months evaporated in that elongated, tortuous moment. I told myself he must be late or sick. I waited there alone for hours, feeling more and more shrinkingly small. All sensations were physical: I had no thoughts. I was emotionally anesthetized. I never saw Big John again. I returned many times, over the summer days, and since in my memories. What the hell happened? The memories remain undiluted to this day, implanted on my shoulders like beleaguered sentries vying to be heard, one whispering longings, the other warnings. I still want to grab Big John's massive arm and tell him, "I did go to college like you said." But this was not to be.

Origins of Loss

I have no conscious memory of ever *not* being tied to loss. Even as a young boy, I felt deeply anchored to loss. Everything deteriorates, gets lost, or simply ends: grandparents die, favorite pajamas are outgrown, Mousketeer Ears fall apart, books get ragged, new immaculate Converse sneakers get their first stain and then wear out, beloved grammar school teachers move on to the next group of eager students. My mother would become gently exasperated with me, "Matthew, where do these thoughts come from? You think too much. Life is beautiful! Go out and play!"

But the realities of loss were very real to me, and this was reinforced by what was going on around me. The aftermath of World War II was everywhere: movies, television, emotionally charged conversations of war stories, and prolonged discussions about its implications. I remember being indoctrinated with multiple messages of nostalgic solidarity: a united country where everyone was equal and of one mind. But all I was seeing were piles of rubble that were formerly gilded European cities. I was indoctrinated with the message that evil wins, a lot. Rather than denying what was so much bigger than what I could integrate—this vulnerability and exposure to danger and death—I absorbed it. I submitted that, like air, random loss and death were nonnegotiable parts of the indivisible fabric of existence.

My father, a World War II veteran, specifically said the Holocaust was allowed to happen because people remained silent. This particular message permeated my consciousness and became an essential element of my evolving character.

Growing up in a four-bedroom apartment with a single bathroom shared by nine people—two parents and seven children—was inherently laden with loss. There was seldom enough of anything: the sense of security that money brings, the unburdened opportunity to be joyful children, time together. My exhausted, work-weary father had little time left for us after working two mindless jobs, from tugboats on the Hudson River and Staten Island Ferry to driving meat delivery trucks in Manhattan. When we did connect, he taught me to love music, read, work hard, and avoid risk.

I have one distinct memory of going to work with him on a tugboat on the overnight shift. There was no romance there. The captain was accepting of my presence but not encouraging: "Stay over there." The benches in the captain's cabin smelled like old, cracked, dirty leather. It was cold, busy, and loud, an uncoordinated and overlapping yet effective symphony of men yelling at each other. I was in awe yet felt so out of place in this water world of real men. I knew then and would share with my mother, "This is not the job for me" and "some of those men said really bad words!" I still wonder if my father brought me there to scare me into getting an education. It worked! But on some level, I sensed that getting an education also meant being different from my family, and that was scary.

I always knew we were poor and it bothered me—a lot. That level of vulnerability was intolerable. I remember asking my father repeatedly if we were middle-class. He would become irritated and say, "No! We are *working* class!" or if really tired, "We are working *poor!*" I felt cut off and suffocated by these words. My mother, who was protective of my father, never spoke about it. Mostly, I felt shame, not so much about being poor, but about the resentment I felt about it.

Although there was a chronic lack of money in my family, cohesiveness, mutual protection, humor, and food were never in short supply. Nor was the revolving door of aunts and uncles who visited us for days or even weeks at a time. Physical space for them did not exist, but it was never a problem or even a question. Intimate space expanded for family. I felt particularly special when my aunts and uncles visited. The men saw it as their sacred mission to (mis)instruct on what a man should *not be* rather than what he *could be*: "don't be a girl," "don't show fear," "don't wait to be hit, punch first, ask questions later," "don't cry, men don't cry." The women were love magicians who praised, hugged, laughed, cooked, and constantly told you how much you were loved.

My mom and dad, despite the zeitgeist and having personally experienced prejudice throughout their lives, believed that all people deserved to be respected and loved, including those who had not earned it. Their courage was linked to personal integrity and honesty. Racism was evil. Racist comments and cursing were simply not tolerated in our home.

I felt protective of, close to, and loved my family. Yet I sensed from an early age there was more to life than what was being lived around me. Compared to my family and friends, I felt left out of a bigger life that I could only hope existed at the other end of the gaseous city buses doubling as rolling advertisements for Brylcreem: "A little dab'll do ya." Thanks to my father, books were always accessible, unlimited passports to anywhere. The more

I read, the greater the intensive drive to participate in those places, to be a part of this assumed yet unknown universe. I was steeped in the life of my family, but my wanderlust for more took me out of that space that could have been more intimate.

Spit It Out Already

In the fifth grade what had once been a very mild stutter became an uncontrollable monster. Early on, I was both fascinated and repulsed by what I imagined would be an unwelcome but transitory visitor. Stuttering meant ordering food I did not want: I desperately chose words I could pronounce, as pointing was not always an option. Telephone calls were even harder given the speed at which I had to get the words out before the recipient might hang up. High school was the worst. Meeting girls in an all-boys Catholic school was hard enough. Stuttering was not high on the list of sought-after characteristics for relationships—or friendships, for that matter.

Paradoxically, giving a speech was not a problem as I could switch words easily, but having casual conversations could be humiliating. Even saying my name could be a real challenge: M's were hard. People often assume that stress impacts stuttering, but stress had little to do with it for me. Stuttering was a spontaneous physical assault upon awaking, a seizure of the throat and neck. I could be at work (where I had to quickly call out arriving/departing trains to the next Penn-Central train tower or, later, while employed at Memorial Sloan-Kettering Cancer Center giving lectures nationally and internationally), on vacation, or enjoying a leisurely day off. The context did not matter. I would wake up in the morning and know immediately if the day would be exhausting. I avoided talking whenever I could get away with it. This was a case where it was much more easily done than said. Many times I was asked, "Are you mentally retarded?" This was a difficult period of rumination, regression, and retreat to books and music. Multiple attempts at speech therapy did not help. Both my confidence and voice were lost. Some mornings, I wished not to wake up.

It would not be until I was forty years old, coinciding with my recruitment to the Johns Hopkins Oncology Center, that dependable fluency returned. A new type of speech therapy focusing on attention and intention to breathing, timing, vibration of vocal folds, and lots of individual and group-focused practice made a significant difference. Slowly, my confident voice returned. I still use these techniques today.

Even now, the memory of stuttering makes me angry and secretly fearful of recurrence. Anger at the losses caused by avoiding situations where having a speaking voice was essential (like almost everywhere); remaining passive in situations where I had something meaningful to add; knowing I was a gifted communicator, but could not be counted on to be fluent on command; and being made fun of by others. Fortunately, the core experience of learning to tolerate vulnerability caused by the lack of trust, control, and reliability over my ability to speak made me stronger. Stuttering reinforced how I felt about life. There is so little I can count on, and even that will probably change at the next relentless swing of the pendulum.

Timefulness: The Fabric That Holds My Life Together

In the early 1970s, when I was nineteen years old, I enrolled at City University of New York and took a job on the Penn-Central Railroad to pay my tuition. I moved into a small, one-bedroom tenement in the Castle Hill section of the Bronx. It was no castle. The apartment was tiny and run down. I did not have hot water in the shower for three years, but that did not stop me from acquiring five fine antique clocks. Living alone for the first time in my life, the quiet was terrifying. The clocks brought me comfort, hope, and musical chimes on the hour. They not only became friends, they were dependable works of art and a connection to something beautiful. I have ten antique clocks now. They serve as a reminder that I am merely the custodian of my time, not the controller.

My building was so close to the elevated part of the Number 6 train that I could almost touch the unevenly painted rusted steel columns from my window. Every ten minutes, during morning and evening rush hours, my apartment shook and rattled in the undeniably nonhuman explosion of an approaching train, in the harmony only cold steel on steel can resonate.

Working on the railroad was my route to paying for college (and eating). I was a towerman and then train director. The trains came into the yard and the same trains went out, same time, same tracks, day after day after day. The work was noisy, stressful, and monotonous, a constant reminder to hit the books or remain a suffocating stationary observer of quicksilver time.

I spent this eight-year period of my life running—exhausted and distracted—from home to school (not Saturday and Sunday), school to work (not Monday and Tuesday), work to home, home to schoolwork. Being in the moment was where I lived, but it was never in the present moment: I was always on the way to the next thing, task, job, assignment, test. Singular focus, emotional isolation, as flexible as steel, reflected the survival plan I created. Other than the few remaining kosher delis and family Italian restaurants, I longed to be anywhere but where I was.

Momma's Boy

I do not remember a time when my mother, Concetta Greco Loscalzo, skinny, short, with dyed fiery-red hair, was not working physically hard: cooking three meals a day for nine people, caring for us, perpetually deep cleaning while hiding how anxious she felt. She suffered from anxiety throughout her short forty-nine years of life. Her love for family, strong religious faith, ubiquitous mile-long cigarettes, and meprobamate (the antianxiety medication of choice at the time) remain the overriding visual for me.

I was deeply connected to my mother. In fact, I was what people called a "Momma's Boy." She liked to talk, and I never ran out of questions. She was upbeat, I was naturally dark. "Why do people die?" "Why do we need to go to the bathroom?" "Why does Grandma (also known as the "Water Buffalo") have so much hair on her face?"

Despite seven kids competing for her attention, my mother somehow made each of us feel uniquely special. "God put me on earth to have babies," she would tell us. My mother seldom complained, but she certainly did worry aloud about her children. Will we be safe and happy? Will we have children? My mother had eight pregnancies but only carried seven to term. However, in her mind, she had eight children and never fully recovered from the loss of her baby. When we two owls spoke late at night, the only quiet time, she would mention that she had a "lost child." Even at a young age, I sensed that, for my mother, this undiminished loss, as physical as well as mental, was a living memory. I would be reminded much later how deep this loss went.

Love, Deception, and Death

In June 1973, one year after finally leaving the housing projects, where she was mugged as a parting gift, and moving to her single-family dream home in Suffolk Country, New York, my mother Concetta Greco Loscalzo died a miserable painful death. I was twenty-one years old.

Unknown to me, this would be the last meeting between my mother and me, one week before her demise. It was also the week I was cramming for final exams.

First, the physical: forty-nine-year-old Caucasian female at home, widely metastatic gastroesophageal cancer, end-stage, pain score 10+ (primarily bone pain in both legs), wasting, emaciated (approximately seventy-five pounds).

In the past, visiting my deteriorating mother was sad, but not torturous. This meeting was different. This time, there would be no love-scolding about how much garlic, pignoli, fresh eggs, raisins, parsley, imported Reggiano parmigiana, but no salt, in the gently browned (not cooked through) meatballs. My mother, once an energetic powerhouse, was now flat on her back, a skeleton lying on top of large black industrial trash bags. The garbage bags reminded me of the containers that prisoners used when cleaning the shoulders of the filthy New York highways. She was mildly delirious, cachectic, writhing in pain, begging me to take wet steaming towels from boiling water on the gas stove and place them on her inflamed, toothpick legs. The pain pills were on the nightstand, just out of reach, like the truth. I made multiple trips to the kitchen to recycle the steaming wet and dripping towels. Too hot to handle, I commandeered two old, large wooden red-stained cooking spoons to keep from getting burned. I was not prepared for what was happening. I felt then, as I do now, that I was torturing her. She thanked me, which only made it worse.

The doctor gave my father two directives: (1) only give my dying mother the oral pain medications he prescribed if absolutely necessary so she would not die addicted and (2) do not take away her hope by telling her the truth. The sailor with a ninth-grade education had his marching orders from his uniformed superior. He blindly followed his orders, and I conveniently and blindly followed mine.

"Am I dying?" Mother asked.

"No. You're going to get better." Her loving son answered.

I went back to the Bronx and to my final examinations vacillating among denial, grief, and lacerating guilt.

Go Say Goodbye to Your Mother

At the end, in my mother's final moments, I was not with her, although the rest of my family was. I arrived at my mother's bedside one hour after she died. In that moment, I also did not realize that she was dead: I thought she was sleeping. When my brother said, "Go say goodbye to your mother," I was confused even further. After touching her, I felt the cold, reflexive shock and heard my internal dialogue: "My mother is gone." I remember my father saying, "She held on as long as she could. Your mother kept looking around the room for you. She knew you were missing." Concetta Greco Loscalzo died searching for another lost child.

Until her last breath, my mother was reassured she would recover, all pain-wracked, dwindling seventy-five pounds of her. Yet we knew she was dying. We all knew that concentration camp look. We, the "courageous" men in her life, believed she was not able to handle the truth. But we were the ones too afraid to handle it. My voice was lost once again. How could I have not remembered that secrecy is fertile ground for evil?

"Am I dying?" I believe now that when my mother asked me if she was dying, what she really meant was: *Matthew, based on our connection and history of conversations, can I talk with you about the fact that I am dying?* I balked and disintegrated. I abandoned her. I was complicit in the lie. She knew she was dying, but she had no one to talk to about it. She could not know she would die alone with this information. As a result, we all suffered major, irreparable loss: not being able to share the sadness of our lives in intimate language unique to a mother and child; not being able to say goodbye; not being able to redefine hope at the end of life within the reality of dying; not being able to stop the physical pain; and, most of all, not protecting each other from the isolation and suffering caused by silence and secrecy.

Although I cannot know for sure what my mother, if given the chance, would have wanted to talk with me about, it almost certainly would have been about family, about having children. I would have told her that I was proud of her, that she was a wonderful mother, and that I loved her deeply. This loss is one of my sins to carry. I hold it close to me. It is a connection to my mother that continues to make me a better person. People who are in my life are treasured, and I try to love them intensely.

I did not know then that losing my mother was something I would never truly get over and would have to work hard to simply get through. True closure for me, and I believe for most others, is a myth. At every milestone, my mother is there with me: my graduations, receiving awards, getting married (not sharing the joy of meeting Joanne), the death of my father at eighty-nine years of age. I carry the accumulated losses of my parents and, since, my older sister (who gave me my Mouseketeer Ears and was a surrogate mother) as precious bridges to the unique connections we shared. Even my sins of the "nots"—not being honest about my mother's dying, not advocating for her pain management, not being there when she died—are connections I will not abandon. Betraying the person who created me, who was my most dependable supporter and fellow dreamer, changed me for the better. It is sad that she had to pay the price for my benefit, yet again.

For over forty years, I have tried to undo and learn from what I will always believe was my loss of integrity during my mother's dying days. Since 1980, I have counseled thousands of cancer patients in pain, women and men, young and old, rich and poor, Asian, Hispanic, Black, Caucasian, all of them connections to my mother. I knew that helping people around small concerns would not be enough for me. Couples arguing over who squeezed the toothpaste from the wrong side of the tube would have been spiritual death for me. I needed to work in situations where the stakes were high. I have always been drawn to the inherent strengths of people, deeply acknowledging what is lost, but only on the way to actively supporting what is left. The connection I value most has been my focus on creating safe spaces for open, compassionate, courageous, and honest communication in real time: *no secrets, no silence.* At times, my reactions have been disproportionate and not very skillful. Still highly prevalent in healthcare today is the "let's try one more (ineffective) treatment" which forestalls the emotionally charged, ethical, compassionate, and courageous conversations that can transform isolated suffering into healing. I keep my "retrospectroscope" at the ready when I sense any slippage into fear and rationalizations.

For me, these emotionally charged memories of loss do not dissipate, disappear, or weaken. They wander around, always at the ready to be reignited. I accept that the world is in constant flux and therefore nothing can be truly counted on, for any of us. Intense loyalty is my personal rage against the

relentless reality of mercurial time. Loss taught me that part of losing included no longer having what is highly valued and, as significantly, accepting
that relationships I wish for may not materialize.

Loss and the need to be resilient have been good preparations for life, albeit with personal costs. With my father, everything was work and had to
be earned. In the end, I am a lot like him: we share this loss, of prioritizing
work above all. The value of hard work was reinforced by my parents, Big
John, and many other experiences in which self-worth was undifferentiated
from work. Being financially secure while living frugally and independently
harkens back to my early feelings of vulnerability about being poor and not
being able to count on anyone to take care of me. I remember the fear on my
parents' faces when they talked about the money they did not have and had
no way of earning. I felt guilty that I had needs and so wanted to help them.
Having these experiences at an early age, I could not allow myself to be that
exposed. Not being successful was never an option.

While the compartmentalizing of work as a sanctuary/escape (learned
from my father and readily imitated by me) and being deeply committed, albeit emotionally controlled, I maintain distance from loved ones. To be much
closer reconnects me to "childhood" feelings of powerlessness in taking care
of those I love and the reality that one day I will lose them.

Still, I am a work in progress. The effort has been more than worth
it. I have been living a truly amazing life, well beyond what I could have
ever realistically imagined. I have used time and loss to become a much
more courageous and loving partner to my wife of twenty years, Joanne
Mortimer, which has deeply enriched my personal life. She deserves and
has a right to expect no less. There is no time to argue over toothpaste
tubes for us. This is a place where my couple's counseling skills have come
back to help me: "When you first decided to be a couple, you knew, in
your core, that the relationship would eventually end. That one of you
would die first. But you had the audacity to commit anyway. This moment in time is a unique opportunity to be proud of how you love and
respect each other."

I have never stopped staring into the face of the stranger in the mirror.
I have noted every new crack and crinkle with surprising resignation. It is
the unstoppable and indisputable fading-in of my father's face that is most
inscrutable. I am more accepting of the long-predicted physical disintegra-
tion than the anticipation of not knowing how low it will go before the breath

departs and lights go out. There comes a certain freedom in knowing I will eventually be forgotten. And, as always, I remain attentive to the precious gift of time. It does not take ten antique clocks to know that time is a fleeting stream, every moment a loss. The clocks are ticking for me and thee, all the time, every day, until they do no longer. I refuse to waste time swimming up the Niagara Falls of inevitable demise. I am having the time of my life until then.

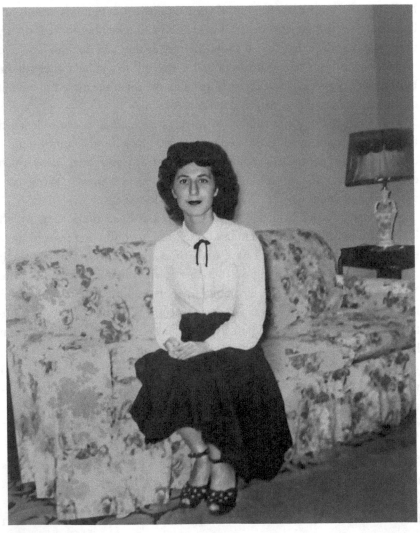

Mom, the only memory I have of her sitting

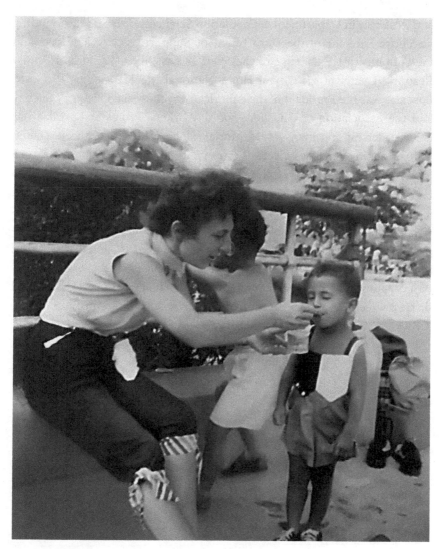

Food, still our connection

About the Author

Matthew Loscalzo, LCSW, APOS Fellow, is an Executive Director, People & Enterprise Transformation Emeritus Professor Supportive Care Medicine, Professor Population Sciences at the City of Hope-National Medical Center. Until August 2021, he was the Liliane Elkins Professor in Supportive Care Programs in the Department of Supportive Care Medicine and Professor in Department of Population Sciences. He is also the founding Executive Director of the Department of Supportive Care Medicine and the Administrative Director of the Sheri & Les Biller Patient and Family Resource Center at the City of Hope–National Medical Center. Professor Loscalzo was the President of the American Psychosocial Oncology Society and the Association of Oncology Social Workers. Professor Loscalzo has held leadership positions at Memorial Sloan-Kettering Cancer Center, Johns Hopkins Oncology Center, Eastern Virginia Medical School, Rebecca and John Moores Cancer Center at the University of California, San Diego (UCSD), and is now in his fourteenth year at City of Hope–. He has been a consultant to multiple major cancer organizations on how to build supportive care programs, implement new processes, and enhance staff engagement and he has developed a unique staff leadership model. His clinical interests and scholarly contributions are gender-based medicine, strengths-based approaches to psychotherapies, pain management, problem-based distress screening, and the creation of supportive care programs.

7

"Did Your Mother Ever Die?"

Fredda Wasserman

There I sat in the hospital waiting room at 3 P.M. on a Sunday afternoon, stunned, disoriented, suspended in disbelief. I was twenty-eight years old, the only child of my precious mama who had not been seriously ill a day in her life. A physician whom I had never met before had just informed me that my mother had died. I wasn't prepared for this news. On the contrary. Only thirty minutes before I had been at her hospital bedside rejoicing over how well she was recovering from her sudden heart attack, which had occurred just three days prior! I vividly recall the myriad of emotional and visceral sensations I experienced during those pivotal seventy-two hours which led up to the moment that changed my life as I knew it.

Thursday: "Your Mother Had a Heart Attack"

Let's start at the beginning.

The saga had begun on what seemed to be quite an ordinary Thursday morning. I tended to my usual responsibilities at the highly respected convalescent hospital where I had done my public health internship and worked for the last half-dozen years as Education Director. I was in the midst of lunch with my colleagues when my husband Bruce showed up at the dining room door. When he beckoned me to join him in the lobby, I stood up, but my muscles locked, and I could not propel myself forward. It must have been the blanched expression on Bruce's face that alerted me that something was wrong, very wrong. Bruce is a man with a calm, soothing presence, always supportive and loving, and it would not be like him to arrive unannounced at my workplace. And I had never seen the intense look of concern that I now saw in his eyes. I felt sick to my stomach. Tentatively, we took a few steps toward each other, and I fell into his arms.

Bruce gently recounted his having received a phone call at work from my father relaying a painful message. "Fredda, your mother had a heart attack this morning. She is in the cardiac unit, and we are leaving right now to get to the hospital." A sense of lightheadedness came over me as I struggled to make sense of Bruce's words. He painstakingly explained that mom had fainted on the bedroom floor at home that morning. Dad called 911, and, when the ambulance arrived, the EMTs wanted to take her to the hospital immediately. But mom was in the middle of her volunteer responsibility editing the monthly newsletter for City of Hope, and she refused to leave the house until she had completed the task. Dad sent the ambulance away, but when Mom collapsed a second time half an hour later, Dad refused to take no for an answer and he drove her to the hospital.

Through a woozy blur, I grabbed my purse and mumbled to my staff that I was leaving. Now we were traveling the familiar 120-mile route from Los Angeles to Palm Springs which Bruce and I had taken innumerable times before for joyful visits. But today we were filled with fear and dread. This being decades before cellphones, we had no way to communicate or get updates along the road. Endless thoughts raced through our minds as we asked each other the unspeakable: "Will she be in pain?" "How weak do you think she will be?" "What if we get there and she has died?" Those were scary thoughts, ones which I may have given voice to on a theoretical level but never actually considered as a *current* possibility. Afterall, Mom and Dad had just stayed with us the previous weekend, when mom spontaneously had an urge to see the updates on our house improvements. She had baked us one of her famous orange chiffon cakes, and Bruce and I were still enjoying little slices of this delicious comfort-food dessert every evening. That was the sweet family life I could relate to. This bewildering new turn of events had no right to cast a shadow on my world, create such inner turmoil, and turn my whole universe upside down!

At last, we arrived at the hospital on that dismal afternoon, and I was startled to find mother sitting up in bed, fully alert, and apologizing for having alarmed us and taken us away from our daily routines. What a strange mixture of surprise and relief I experienced. Much of the foreboding panic I had been feeling dissipated. Mom insisted that we *not* notify the extended family who lived out of town because she would be home in no time and wanted no cards, flowers, or visitors. Just us.

Throughout the day, the medical team continued to give us positive updates. We were convinced that this episode would turn out to be just a blip in Mom's medical history, most likely requiring her to make some minor changes in her diet, perhaps move from their upstairs condo to a ground floor unit, and stop smoking. The latter would be a welcome change. From the time I was a little girl, I despised the smell of cigarettes in the house and in the car, and, when I grew up, I had forbidden my parents to smoke in my apartment. Yet in those days there was much less emphasis on the health risks involved with smoking, and I had not considered her to be putting her life in danger by continuing this life-long habit. How naïve. I now recognize that I had been brainwashed by watching years of ads on TV touting her brand of cigarettes. I distinctly remember as a child proudly presenting my mother, more than once, with a hand-painted clay ashtray as a holiday "gift." But here I digress.

Friday: "I Hope That We Will Have Daughters, Mom"

Because mom was doing so well, I supported Bruce in his decision to drive round-trip back to Los Angeles to fulfill his Saturday morning commitment to seeing his own patients at his medical clinic. That left me and dad alone for the evening. This might have given us a chance to have a meaningful father–daughter talk; however, characteristic of our relationship, we spoke very little and kept our feelings to ourselves. Dad had never been very good about expressing his emotions, other than with tears. The first time I saw my Dad cry was when my grandfather died. My being only seven or eight at the time, it frightened me to see him behave in this unfamiliar manner. Dad flew back east the next morning to attend the funeral, but he never spoke to me about it. When I was in high school, my dad's eyes welled up whenever I sang his favorite song "Sunrise, Sunset." I saw the smile behind the tears in his eyes as I walked across the stage at my graduation and at my wedding. But he was consistently a man of few words. Illness and death were definitely not topics my father was comfortable discussing. I even remember Mom once telling me that my Dad had never purchased medical insurance. Can you believe it? He did not have medical insurance because he thought it might bring bad luck. Perhaps this magical thinking protected him from having to feel scary or painful feelings. Once, when he overheard Mom and me having a heartfelt conversation about death, he stood up and walked out of the room saying, "Why talk about that?"

So unlike the relationship with Mom. She and I had closeness and an effortless rapport, whether we were talking about the events of our daily lives, making plans for upcoming visits, or just enjoying each other's presence without having to talk at all. I always felt deeply connected to Mom on an energetic level. We loved being mother and daughter! And our intimate conversations continued throughout her hospital stay.

I have often reflected on one conversation in particular. Although Bruce and I had been married for seven years, we had not felt ready to have children. And it was a subject that my parents respectfully never inquired about. I didn't mention to her that day that I had just gone off birth control pills and would soon be trying to get pregnant. I am grateful that I *did* tell her that Bruce and I had discussed having two children, and, unlike my cousin who had two boys, "I hope that we will have daughters, Mom, I want to be able to share experiences with them, like we do." That's as close as she came to hearing that she would someday have grandchildren.

Saturday: "Let's Have Breakfast"

Those few days, I was essentially living in a cocoon, insulated from the outside world. Staying in the condo with my Dad and having told no one what was going on with my mother's health made it even more unreal. I did remind myself to maintain my routine of eating, sleeping, and exercising, but everything else was out of the ordinary. While I was swimming laps the next morning, my heart jumped into my throat when I heard Dad calling to me from his balcony. I darted out of the pool and into the condo, anticipating some very bad news, only to have Dad say "Let's have breakfast." There I went again, riding the emotional rollercoaster that oscillated between the mundane and the unfathomable. I was visiting my parents, but there was only one parent home. It was time for breakfast, but Mom wasn't there to nourish us with one of her delicious meals. I was the child, but I was being asked to fulfill my mother's role. I had always been aware that Mom had nurtured and taken care of Dad throughout their life together. Now he was turning to me to be attentive to what he needed. Dad was a wonderful provider, but not a nurturer. I accepted that this was how he was without giving it too much conscious thought, although I was craving a little more parenting. Internally, I was crying out to be taken care of. After downing our French toast, Dad and I headed to the shopping mall to attend to more practical needs. I purchased a change of clothes since, with the suddenness of our departure, I had not had a chance to pack a bag. Ironically, I felt good in the outfit that day, but I was never in the mood to wear it again. The navy and white boat-necked sweater and uncomfortable slacks themselves evoked too many memories of those ill-fated days when everything felt out of place, and my life was changing at a warped speed.

We spent Saturday afternoon visiting our ever-optimistic patient in the antiseptic environment of the CCU. Seeing Mom propped up in a bed, wearing a general-issue medical gown, and hearing the irritating beeps of the cardiac monitors was both unfamiliar and unpleasant. This was so different from the nurturing atmosphere she cultivated in her home, where I always felt cozy and soothed. To this day, I can sense that cuddly feeling in my body when I picture being a child sitting with Mom on our living room couch after dinner, Mom peeling an orange or cutting apple slices and serving it with sugar cookies as a TV snack. It was incongruous visiting and then leaving her here in the hospital. We kissed her, went to dinner, and made it through another night.

Sunday: "We Were Unsuccessful"

On Sunday morning they moved Mom from the cardiac unit to a private room on the medical floor. We were greatly encouraged by this and felt certain she was out of the woods. Bruce and I stopped at a local florist on the way to see her and presented Mom with a hand-selected floral bouquet and a whimsical rabbit puppet on a stick that popped up out of a cylinder. There were lots of smiles and hugs. When the doctor came in to make his rounds, Bruce, my dad, and I decided to take a walk around the hospital gardens. We took our time, admiring the flower beds and enjoying the warm desert air. I was so grateful that Mom was getting better, and my mind was caught up with making plans for taking her back home and how we would visit in the weeks ahead. Enough of this hospital business! I was oblivious to the presence of the security guard nearby and the voice emitting from his walkie-talkie "code blue, code blue, second floor." Bruce would tell me weeks later that he froze when he heard those words. I imagine that even if I had been tuned in to the announcement, no way would I have speculated that it was my mother who was in distress.

Upon re-entering the building, my father headed straight to Mom's room. Bruce and I found our way up to the library and peered down over the railing into the central courtyard. Suddenly a blood-curdling shriek reverberated through the atrium and echoed in my ears. It sounded like my Dad screaming "Fredda." We bolted for the stairwell, descended several flights, and found my Dad sitting in a tiny waiting area, crying hysterically. A fog of numbness set in as the doctor explained in somber tones, "Your mother had a second heart attack; we tried everything, but we were unsuccessful." I felt like a little girl, frightened, naïve, and powerless, silently shaking my head in dissent, my mind protesting the message he was imparting. When I finally spoke, with imperfect grammar I asked him, "Did your mother ever die?"

"No, but my father did," he calmly replied. Hearing the physician answer in such an honest manner, for a very brief moment I felt strangely comforted that I wasn't the only one. Someone else close to my age, this man who could not have been more than a few years older than me, knew what I was feeling. I hadn't known anyone else who had had a parent die. I was suddenly plunged into unknown territory where I did not recognize my surroundings or even myself. Out of the blue, I had become motherless.

I wanted to see her. The doctor held my arm so that I didn't crumple into a heap on the floor and walked me toward her room. There I stood, peering in from the partially open doorway. Once again, I became paralyzed and unable to move; my eyes transfixed on her uncharacteristically distended stomach and her motionless body. Such a stark contrast to my mother's ordinarily animated self. This time there was no turning toward me, breaking into a big smile, or greeting me with the familiar, "Hi, Sweetie." Would I never hear those words again? My head was spinning. I was overcome by a dysphoria that filled me with a combination of anxiety and confusion. Somehow, although I could still see her lying there, Mom's life-force was gone. I did not want this to be true. I wanted to shout, "Mama, where are you?" but I remained numbly silent. I could not bear to get any closer, and I staggered away in a daze from this disconcerting scene.

Ready to leave the hospital, but too physically and emotionally exhausted to drive, we called my aunt and uncle. I heard Bruce succinctly relating the essential facts of the past three days: "Irene had a heart attack on Thursday; we all thought she was improving, but she had a second one today. She died just a few minutes ago." He asked that they pick us up and take us home with them. We could not face going back into Mom and Dad's house. My father, unable to speak through his sobs, sat beside his sister and didn't move for hours. I was adamant that it was my excruciating responsibility to call all the aunts and uncles around the country to tell them that Mom had died. One by one, I dialed their numbers. I was OK explaining her heart attack, but from there I fell into using more cryptic language: "Today, well, you know . . ." or "You have to come." I could not yet say the word "died."

I spent a virtually sleepless night thrashing around in bed, dozing off occasionally and then being jolted awake by the sinking reality that the unthinkable had happened. *My mother was dead.* My mother. The woman who had so openly and honestly guided me through all of life's passages. The personification of emotional intelligence and wisdom. She had explained to me at the age of eight that our neighbor, Mrs. Larson, would probably have a hard Christmas that year, given that it would be the first holiday since her mother's death. The nurturing mama who I had watched comfort my Dad when his father died. And now I was suddenly and unexpectedly thrust into this role of making funeral plans and decisions about shiva and mourning rituals without her. And *for* her.

Monday: "Maybe This Can Be Just a Bad Dream"

We briefly stopped at Mom and Dad's—was it still her house now that she had died? We grabbed a few essentials and began the two-hour drive home from Palm Springs. It was tortuous. My father wailed in the back seat as I silently stared at the road ahead like a zombie. Cars whizzed by. Traffic sounds were muffled. People in other cars appeared to be going about their everyday lives. But inside of me nothing made sense; everything was happening in slow motion.

Close relatives were already in the living room when I entered my house. However, rather than sit and converse with them, I started cleaning. No matter how they beseeched me, "*Sit down, Fredda, have a bite to eat, drink some water,*" I was unable to comply. My mind was racing; maybe if I kept moving the pain would go away and all of this would be just a bad dream.

Thank goodness my parents had settled on their burial arrangements years before. In fact, I had gone to the cemetery with them many times to visit the graves of my grandparents and Mom and Dad's own "real estate," as they jokingly referred to the plots where they would someday be buried alongside three aunts and uncles. Now that time had arrived. There were very few decisions to be made when we met with the memorial counselor that afternoon. Still, it took several hours to finalize all the details. Walking into the casket room to approve the latest model of the coffin was about as surreal as it could get. In that moment, I distinctly remembered my Mom describing how she almost fainted when she went in to make her choice and pictured herself nestled into the satin lining.

Tuesday: "What Do You Think Friends Are For?"

On the day of the funeral, my state of shock was compounded by being driven to the cemetery in a limousine, seeing the name "Irene Avidon" on the signboard outside the sanctuary, and having to identify my mother's body. Yes, that was her. I had hastily, though wisely, chosen for her to be buried in the dress she wore on my wedding day. It brought sweet memories to this tragic scenario. I smiled and cried as I gazed down at her lifeless body. She was beautiful, as she always was to me. Her hair was perfectly coiffed, but the lipstick color was all wrong. She wore orange, not pink! How was I to know that I should have brought along her own makeup and a photo?

Promptly at eleven, the usher directed us to take our places seated behind a curtain. I felt like I was on autopilot or playing a role in a film as the composed daughter, assuring that everyone in attendance was well taken care of and things were running smoothly. Internally, I was devastated by the ache and emptiness in my chest and reeling from the swirling in my head. The rabbi began the prayers and eulogy. He recited the poem "Woman of Valor," with which I was not acquainted. The line "Her worth is far beyond rubies" was tailor-made for Mom, as the ruby was her birthstone.

Friends and family came up to us after the service and offered words of consolation. But nothing could have soothed my anguish on that day. On one hand, I was touched by how many people from all walks of my mother's life had come to honor her memory. Yet I was irritated by one woman whom I had not seen for years when she whipped out a small picture album and called out "Come here, Fredda, I want you to see pictures of my newborn granddaughter. Isn't she adorable?" I wanted to bite her head off. Did she think this was some kind of festive get-together?

My best friend and her Mom really got it when they offered to hard boil dozens of eggs and stay at my house during the service and burial to set up the reception and receive the food that was being delivered. I expressed my amazement that they would take on this responsibility when they, too, had experienced a great loss and were in a state of grief. When I thanked them profusely at the end of the day, my friend's mother held my face in her hands, looked into my eyes, and asked in a choked voice, *"What do you think friends are for, just coming to parties?"* With those words, they taught me that *is* what friends are for; as the song says, to be there in good times and bad times.

Throughout the weeks and months that followed, 3 A.M. became the quintessential hour for expression of my grief. I felt so depleted in every way most days that I fell immediately into a deep sleep the minute my head hit the pillow. And then I would bolt awake at three. After the initial confusion, during which everything seemed OK for a few seconds, the reality would hit. This was not just a bad dream; that pit in my stomach and the uncontrollable, relentless tears plunged me deeply into the abyss of loss and grief. It was those middle-of-the-night awakenings, when I needed to be held and soothed, that I was most grateful for Bruce's being so attuned to my emotions. I distinctly remember feeling that my heart had been cracked open. And still, through it all, I was aware that while the pain was enormous, there was something I liked about the rawness and real-ness of being connected to my Mom through the depth and genuineness of these sensations.

My father, on the other hand, was not sensitive to my fragile state. It was as if he believed that the person who died was solely his wife, not *my mother*. Not once in the twenty-two years that he lived after Mom's death did he ever ask me how I was feeling or make any mention that he empathized with what I was going through. That was hurtful. I had lost one parent; couldn't my Dad have tried to nurture me like she would have? Yet somehow, I took it in stride, acknowledging that he had never been comfortable talking about feelings. It is only now, as I look back all these years later, that I can see that in his own way he, too, was teaching me about death and grief as I witnessed firsthand the devastation he was experiencing. I now feel grateful for that preparation which he unknowingly imparted to me. He gave me an up close and personal view into the emotions of the grievers who would someday be my clients. Today, when I work with someone like my Dad, I am tolerant of their sometimes limited ability to put their feelings into words. I can sit with them in silence when they cry, and cry, and cry, and not expect that they will be able to describe what is going on for them internally. Reciprocally, these patients have given me an increased compassion for my Dad as I reflect on his myopic perspective when he could only see how Mom's death affected him and not how I was suffering. I empathize with the grown children who are in the position of grieving the death of their Mom or Dad while at the same time shouldering the responsibility of caring for their surviving parent.

I accepted my Dad for who he was after Mom died, and I did not get upset with him for forgetting my wedding anniversary, which fell just a few weeks later. And I knew to be prepared for the big events throughout the year. I got through Mother's Day and her birthday reasonably well. It was those everyday moments, when I wanted to pick up the phone to tell her about something I was doing or ask her advice, that I missed her the most. She had always understood how I was feeling and knew just how to respond in her loving, empathetic manner. One day when I was yearning for her companionship, I was profoundly struck by the realization that Mom would have been the one person who could have best consoled me as I coped with her death. Just when I needed her most, she was no longer here.

Of course, there had been other goodbyes. There was the emotional farewell when my parents dropped me off at UC Berkeley and headed home after adding a few personal touches to my dorm room. But that was a planned goodbye, and it was softened by the note Mom had left on my bed addressed "To our CAL GIRL." And the jubilant bon voyage as Bruce and I left for our honeymoon. The letter we received at the hotel that week began with the words, "PERFECT, PERFECT!!!" as she conveyed her over-the-top delight with our wedding day. But this time was different. This goodbye was forever. There was no love note from Mom now. The presence of her absence was glaring.

My grief continued to blindside me, at first every day and then gradually less frequently. And when days or eventually weeks would pass between acute waves of sorrow, I was mystified that my heart was starting to heal. Nevertheless, each year, even after more than a decade, I would find myself weepy, anxious, and out of sorts for no apparent reason at the end of February. Only to become aware that it was just a week before March 6 and the marking of another year. And I would re-live every moment of every day from the time she had her heart attack until the shiva was over. I could feel it viscerally, through each of my senses. The visuals, the smells, the sounds, and most of all the heartache which at times arose as intensely as ever.

"Your mommy died, but she is still your mommy."

Over time I came to recognize new perspectives about my Mom's death, my grief, and the impact and influence she has had on my adult life. I had always appreciated the fact that Mom had delighted in how happily married I was and had cultivated a great relationship with us, filled with mutual caring and peppered with playfulness. But she died before my daughters were born, and I missed her dearly when I became pregnant. How I would have loved to share this news with her! Remembering that she and my Dad had waited 10 years before I was born, I now wondered about her decision to become a mother. There were so many questions about parenthood that I had never asked. I had seen her tender interactions with my cousins' children, but I had to be content with just fantasizing about how she would be with mine. I can only imagine how she would have adored them. I patterned myself after my mother's maternal style as best I could. Like her, I did not work outside the home while raising my children and devoted myself to volunteerism that supported my children's interests as well as the community at large. We both placed a high priority on honesty and openness in our communications.

Mom had taught me about death and grief in the same gentle way that she explained how babies are made—I was the first kid on my block to know the truth about that, too! My mother and I visited the homes of friends and family when a baby was born, attended memorials, and paid condolence calls as loving demonstrations of our appreciation for life's beginnings and endings. I followed in Mom's footsteps when I discussed death openly with my own daughters as they were growing up. When my elder daughter was only three years old and saw me weeping, I explained that I was thinking about my mommy and missing her. "It's ok. Your mommy died, but she is still your mommy," she reminded me. I was making her comfortable with death, just as her grandmother had done for me.

To this day, I carry on Mom's traditions and stay closely connected to her memory in conscious and unconscious ways. When I attend a significant family event that she would have attended had she been alive, I wear her wedding band on my right hand to symbolically have her there with me. When I host a summer party for the extended family, I recall the great pleasure she found in bringing everyone together for annual Chanukah celebrations. When a relative comments that my facial expression or hand gestures remind them of my Mom, my eyes fill with tears . . . happy tears. When I make Mom's chicken soup and brisket recipes and the house smells like Irene's, the evoked memories are bittersweet.

Smiles and tears ebb and flow. When my younger daughter wants to know what Grandma Irene was like, I am only too happy to share memories of everything from playing paper dolls together to being taught how to cook, knit, and crochet. When she cries about missing my in-laws, the grandparents who she knew so well and were such a vital part of her life, I ache, as I wonder what kind of a grandma my Mom would have been to her. When my older daughter was about to be married, heartwarming memories of planning my wedding with Mom were reawakened. I remembered the joy and excitement we had shared when we found my wedding gown, designed a heart-shaped *chuppah* canopy covered with iris and yellow roses, and selected the music. As I became the mother of the bride, I wished my Mom could be here to reminisce with me and be part of this family celebration.

"You Are 28 . . . but Your Mama Didn't Die"

Sometimes history repeats itself in unexpected ways. On a Thursday morning, when my younger daughter was twenty-eight years old, I had a sudden heart attack. I had awakened early that morning with excruciating pain across my upper back; like nothing I had ever felt before. I was short of breath and scared. Unlike my mother, I immediately concluded that I needed to go the emergency room. Bruce called the ER and alerted them to be ready for me. All the compulsory tests were administered, and the diagnosis of a mild heart attack was confirmed. When the cardiologist explained that I was scheduled for an angiogram the following morning, I asked in all seriousness if I could go to the Hollywood Bowl that evening as planned and come back for the procedure the next day. Of course, they would not allow this. As I look back, I realize just how much I reacted as my mother had: I, too, wanted to carry on with my normal life; I, too, believed that I was just fine, with no need to think of myself as a patient. Like my Mom, I was hospitalized for three days. But, unlike her, stents were inserted into my coronary arteries, and I survived. Upon arriving home on Sunday, I said to my daughter, *"You are twenty-eight, and your mama had a heart attack on a Thursday morning, but your mama didn't die."* We held each other and cried.

"Mom, Are You Aware of the Lasting, Positive Impact You Have Had on the Woman I Have Become?"

It is no coincidence that my professional path has led me to develop a psychotherapy practice focusing on end of life and grief. I am honored to bear witness to my clients' experiences and share the intimacy of their journeys. When a patient is facing their own death, or when a griever cannot see that there will ever be light in the world again, I get it. I am often taken back to my own grief, and it opens my heart and allows me to be with them with a sense of compassion and serenity. I am perpetually grateful for my mother having blazed the trail to what has become the most heart-centered career I could ever have imagined.

In a society where life goes on avoiding the topics relating to loss, I am relentless in encouraging intimate conversations about end of life and death among family, friends, patients, and colleagues. This determination motivated me to educate thousands of physicians, medical and nursing students, social workers, educators, and clergy throughout my twenty-year career as Clinical Director of Adult Programs at OUR HOUSE Grief Support Center. It inspired me to co-author with Norine Dresser *Saying Goodbye to Someone You Love: The Emotional Journey Through End of Life and Grief*, and portions of this chapter were adapted from that (Demos Health Publishers, 2010).

The interface between my personal life and work life is exemplified by the exquisite timing of my mother's death occurring just when I was coordinating a course on Elisabeth Kubler-Ross's seminal work on death and dying. I was fully aware of the synchronicity of these occurrences. It seemed as if my mother's life-long modeling, combined with the heart-wrenching experience of losing her, was guiding me forward on this compelling path. It certainly influenced the level of comfort and intimacy I experienced in working with

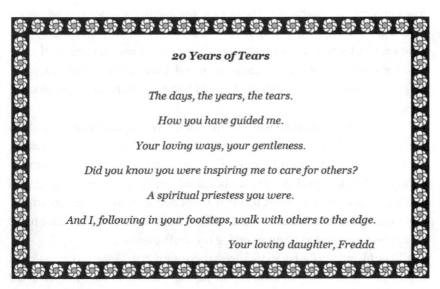

20 Years of Tears

The days, the years, the tears.

How you have guided me.

Your loving ways, your gentleness.

Did you know you were inspiring me to care for others?

A spiritual priestess you were.

And I, following in your footsteps, walk with others to the edge.

Your loving daughter, Fredda

20 Years of Tears

the AIDS community during the 1980s and '90s. I readily paid it forward and bestowed upon my patients the type of loving acceptance and compassion I had gotten from my mother, which they all too often did not receive from theirs.

While writing and editing this chapter, I unexpectedly came across a poem I had written twenty-four years ago on marking the twentieth year since Mom's death. Finding it brought a smile to my face and a warmth to my heart.

I am often asked if doing this work makes it any easier when someone dear to me dies. My immediate answer is "No, it does not." However, I am aware that there are both yes and no responses to this question. On one hand, I *can* answer "Yes." In left-brained, pragmatic ways, I believe that my work did prepare me for the inevitability of death. I long ago accepted the fact that at the end of each life . . . at the very, very end . . . the person dies. And perhaps because of that I never went to the place of asking "Why me?" Or "How could this happen?"

On the other hand, I am much more of a right-brained person. In my world, no amount of knowledge, understanding, or experience in being around death alleviates my deep sadness when someone dear to me dies. It certainly did not make my mother's death any less excruciating on a heart, soul, and feeling level.

Balancing the logical and the emotional led me onto a spiritual/existential path. I discovered ways to both live and grieve as I integrated my mother's death into my life's narrative. Today I am the age my mother was when she died. It is an unsettling feeling to have outlived her. I felt vulnerable when I had my heart attack and came face-to-face with my own mortality. No way did I feel ready to have my life come to an end. I wanted to bargain for more time . . . but with whom? And what would I give in return for being granted a longer life?

I sometimes contemplate why it is that I survived my heart attack and am receiving the gift of years of life that my mother did not get. I have reflected on the question "What do I think of as a full lifetime?" Do I measure life merely in chronological years? I do not think so; yet if I knew I was imminently dying, I know I would feel that I was being cheated. I'm too young. I have more love that I want to share with my family and friends. I have more to experience. I want to go on pursuing my soul's passion.

If I could magically have a conversation with my Mom today, I would begin with: "*Mom, are you aware of the lasting, positive impact you have had on the woman I have become?"* I would be curious to know from her if she believes that her soul accomplished its spiritual purpose. I do not ever remember hearing her speak in such philosophical terms, although one conversation we had reminds me how she accepted the reality of the cycle of life.

About three years before she died, we gave my parents a surprise anniversary party. Mom was overwhelmed by the unexpected presence of her dearest friends and closet relatives giving them a standing ovation as she and Dad entered the restaurant. The next morning, over coffee, with tears in her eyes, Mom expressed her gratitude. "If I died tomorrow, I would die happy. I have had the most wonderful life." Even in the midst of her greatest joy, she remained aware of impermanence.

"Hi, Sweetie"

I know that no matter how many years I have ahead of me, there will be no trophy for who lived the longest. Like my mother, what makes my life meaningful are the experiences and relationships that nurture me. I will always long for one more hug, one more conversation, one more opportunity to be with my mother and hear her say *"Hi, Sweetie."* And at the same time, I maintain a close, loving connection to her memory, I feel her with me, and she continues to enrich my life.

About the Author

Fredda Wasserman, MA, MPH, LMFT, specializes in the healing connection between mind, body, heart, and soul in her work with people who are diagnosed with life-changing illness, those who are grieving, and those who are going through transition in their lives. She received her masters in health education and health administration from the UCLA School of Public Health and her masters in clinical psychology from Antioch University. Fredda is the former Clinical Director of Adult Programs at OUR HOUSE Grief Support Center, where she developed educational programs for medical and mental health professionals, educators, and clergy and was the 2011 recipient of the OUR HOUSE Founder's Award. She is the co-author with Norine Dresser of

Saying Goodbye to Someone You Love: Your Emotional Journey Through End of Life and Grief. Recognized as an expert in death, dying, and bereavement, Fredda has devoted her career to life's final chapter.

Suggested Resources

Dresser, Norine, and Fredda Wasserman. (2010). *Saying goodbye to someone you love: Your emotional journey through end of life and grief.* New York: DemosHealth.

Kessler, David. (2019). *Finding meaning: The sixth stage of grief.* New York: Scribner.

8

Panel 19, Number 9, East

In Memoriam to Larry Insel, 01 May 1967

Mitch Golant

On my first trip to Washington, DC, in 1993, I squeezed in a day of sightseeing between my meetings and conferences. When I came upon the Vietnam War Memorial, I was suddenly seized with the urge to find the name of a long-lost high school friend—Larry—the scion of a prominent family in Los Angeles. This poem came to me as I sat in the Metro train, making my way back to the hotel outside Baltimore. I scribbled it on the back of an envelope. The Vietnam Era shaped my life. Because of the lottery, my friends and I all struggled to find ways to avoid fighting a war we didn't believe in. Threatened with being drafted, I became a teacher in South Central Los Angeles (considered a poverty area), which might have qualified me for a deferment. Eventually, in 1968, I volunteered for a unit in the Reserves, but, to my shock, I failed the physical. Larry's decision to join the armed forces early on stood in contrast to the angst and struggles the rest of our close friends experienced.

My college years were a time of huge social disruption, racial conflict, mistrust of government and its leaders. Anger about the war and racism ran high. Many of the returning vets were scorned and rejected. As we know, some suffered from undiagnosed posttraumatic stress disorder (PTSD), alcoholism, and especially drug abuse. Without adequate support or compassion, many died from illness, drugs, or suicide after returning to the United States. Others ended up homeless on the streets where they still live today.

My sense of loss during the Vietnam War years echoes today's COVID-19 era tragedy. Then and now, there are so many losses: not just relatives and friends, but also the loss of a unified voice of comfort in the face of profound polarities, the persistent lack of civility in public discourse, and the uncertainty—and at times terror—that we all collectively face.

After I visited the Vietnam Memorial, I reached out to Larry's family to let them know that I had remembered him and them. They needed no reminders. I could feel that my call was an intrusion.

I wonder if the poem might speak to a generation of loss yet to come—a cautionary tale of our not-too-distant future.

PANEL 19, NUMBER 9, EAST
IN MEMORIAM TO LARRY INSEL
01 MAY 1967

Mitch Golant, Ph.D. © 1997

Memory of
Olds *Rocket 88*
Smell of
Burning Rubber
Horn Honking
(*"Your horn blows
how about your wife?"*)
No need to knock
Door slamming
In a patch of smoke
and we are
gone—
Laughing all
the way.

At the Modern Day
Wailing Wall—
Searching among
names
Swimming in
Black ink,
All the souls
Cresting in
the sea
Of

Names
Towards
Panel
19
Number
9
East.

(*The last time*
I Saw you) . . .
Spaced out
but
Going To War.

I'm eating a
Bean Burrito
(2 for 45 cents)
You're
Smoking Winstons
Sipping a Coke—two straws
Blowing Smoke
Rings.
Straw paper wrappers
Folded
Accordion-like
Ready to jump
ship
but
dissolve into
A puddle
of
Ice
Chips.
Lost and
Scared:
"Got to go, now." He says.
"Why ya goin'?" I say.

"Nothin' else to do
or be."

55 T-Bird
(*No Portholes.*)
Re-painted
Metallic Gold
Black tuck-and-roll inside
Driving down Olympic Boulevard
Back from Tee's, Sorrento, and Will Rogers
Looking for girls
(In our dreams!)
If only I'd known
Then.
I basking
In your
Clint Eastwood-Kookie-James Dean
Pose.
(I could pass
'Cause you
could Posture).
If only I had known
Then,
What I know
Now.

Standing at the Wall:
Black
On Black
In Black,
Sea of Names
Touching
Searching
Swallowing names like
As a child swallowing
Ocean Water.

Waiting, watching
Hoping to find you . . .
Instead
Seeing
A Vet standing alone
Face pocked and lined
Shivering
Shaking . . .
And Remembering
Rain pouring all over
Running down his back,
Neck,
Penetrating sinew,
Soaking
Everything with Memories.
Staring . . .
Alone
Surrounded by a vision:
Shadow Boxing
Shadow Dancing
Nightmare Holograms
Playing
I turn away
In shame
And look for you
Seeking Solace
In the Black Wall of Names
Waiting to merge
With this
Wailing Wall
Of our youth
To Forget and
Be Forgiven
And
Be One
With it All
Again.

Later,
I see Him
Again.
Waiting,
A Friend's Arm
Wrapped around him.
He,
Draped in green,
Staring . . .
Re-runs playing on the
Screen beyond tears
And rain
Watching and seeing
It
All Again.
And I wonder,
In my heart
"Larry?
Larry . . .
Is
That
You
He
Sees?"

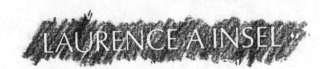

Figure 8.1 Vietnam Veterans Memorial

About the Author

Mitch Golant, PhD, is a health psychologist in clinical practice and Senior Consultant, Strategic Initiatives for the Cancer Support Community (CSC). From 1996 to 2012, he was CSC's Senior Vice-President of Research and Training. In that capacity, he co-founded CSC's Cancer Survivorship Research and Training Institute in Philadelphia, Pennsylvania. He is recognized as a pioneer in the use of information technology in cancer education and support through the delivery of online support groups. He has served on the Board of Directors of the American Psychosocial Oncology Society. In 2011, he received the Los Angeles County Psychological Association's Distinguished Contribution to the Profession of Psychology Award. In 2015, he was elected as a Fellow of the American Psychosocial Oncology Society and received CSC's Harold H. Benjamin Innovation Award. He has co-authored seven books including *Reclaiming Your Life After Diagnosis: The Cancer Support Community Handbook* (BenBella) (2012), *What to Do When Someone You Love Is Depressed* (Holt) (2007), the *Psycho-Oncology Quick Reference Guides in Cancer Symptom Management in Adult and Pediatric Cancer* (2006, 2008, 2014). He is a contributing author of *Psycho-Oncology*, 4th edition (Oxford).

9

Five Decades

Steven T. Rosen

She left the morning of our forty-sixth anniversary
A poignant affirmation of seething anger
Four children, an exquisite granddaughter, hundreds of devoted
friends, a dozen dogs of varied breeds, a quarter horse and
Palomino, eighteen homes, three RVs of assorted lengths, cross
country and global travel, scores of social events, classic movies,
shows and countless sporting contests, beach and mountain
hikes, ten thousand blissful memories and three decades of
supporting her father—all now meaningless commodities
My punishment for all her disappointments in life
Unconditional love an empty anchor no longer valued
Hopefully she will at least remember that
I held her in my arms every night
　　　　　　　　　　　—Steven T. Rosen, *Heartfelt Reflections* (2021)

About the Author

Steven T. Rosen, MD, FACP, FASCO, is Provost, Chief Scientific Officer, and Director of the Comprehensive Cancer Center and the Beckman Research Institute, Irell & Manella Cancer Center Director's Distinguished Chair for the City of Hope in Duarte, California. Following his graduation with distinction from Northwestern University Medical School's Six-Year Honors Program in Chicago, Dr. Rosen completed his residency in internal medicine at Northwestern and a fellowship in medical oncology at the National Cancer Institute (NCI). He served as the Director of the Robert H. Lurie Comprehensive Cancer Center at Northwestern University Feinberg School of Medicine from 1989 to 2014. Dr. Rosen has received numerous grant awards and contracts and has published more than 400 scientific papers. Dr. Rosen's laboratory research focuses on experimental therapeutics and hematologic malignancies. Dr. Rosen is the former chair of the Medical Science Committee of the Leukemia and Lymphoma Society and serves on its Board. He also serves on the Board of American Society of Clinical Oncology's Conquer Cancer Foundation. Dr. Rosen has been an advisor to more than two dozen NCI Comprehensive Cancer Centers. Dr. Rosen has received multiple awards for excellence in science and unwavering commitment to providing compassionate expertise to all patients and their families.

10

Lost and Found

Susan D. Block

I had a lucky life until I was in my late fifties and then, suddenly, a sequence of heartbreaks had me moving through what felt like one long tunnel of loss, with very little rest or respite.

My story starts when my husband of twenty-seven years, Andy, and I were settled into our empty nest: our children were out of the house, and now it was just the two of us. Andy was tall, elegant-looking, serious, moody, literate, had a great sense of humor, and was one of the best listeners I have ever known. After our youngest son went to college, we moved to a smaller house in Harvard Square because we felt isolated from each other in the larger house, where we rattled around in too much space. We loved the coziness and warmth and connectedness we felt in the new house. We shared an office and often worked at our desks together—Andy's desk was large and practical—stacked with papers and books and full of electronic gadgets and assorted whimsical objects; mine, a gift from Andy, was small, beautiful, and much-loved by me, but in real life not very practical.

Our kids were finding their ways in the world: our older son, Josh, was working on his dissertation in classics at Oxford University in the UK, and our younger son, Gabe, a recent college graduate, was on his way to graduate school in physics at Stanford. We were in good health, had a wonderful group of close friends, a strong network of mutual friend-colleagues, and few worries.

We were also both in the midst of meaningful and demanding work, both collaboratively and independently. We had both been leaders in creating the field of palliative medicine in the United States and in educating thousands of clinicians. Andy was the Chief of Palliative Care at Massachusetts General Hospital, and I had just become the Chair of a newly created Department of Psychosocial Oncology and Palliative Care at Dana-Farber Cancer Institute and Brigham and Women's Hospital. We jointly directed the Harvard Medical School Center for Palliative Care, running national and international educational programs in this emerging field. We were pretty driven, worked intensively together on writing projects and teaching, and recognized the synergies we brought to our process.

Andy was more cerebral, methodical, and perfectionistic. I was—and remain—more pragmatic, impatient, and willing to take risks. Because of these differences in our personalities and the strong overlap in our work lives and professional interests, we also had to negotiate issues of control and competition with each other: over our different ideas about how to run our courses, over our leadership styles and their impact on our programs, and over our individual needs for affirmation and recognition. In spite of these challenges, all in all, we had a lucky life, and we knew it.

Then one morning I walked into the kitchen and found nearly every drawer and cabinet open. This was the beginning of a hypomanic episode and its residua that evolved and lasted for two years. I will not say more about it because that is Andy's story and not mine, although it had profound effects on me and on our family.

As Andy stabilized and began to process what had happened, first within himself and then with me and the kids, life began to settle down again. The process was very slow and took many months. The bipolar diagnosis and the medications that finally offered help somehow made it easier for him to accept what had happened. He, and we, experienced great relief that there was finally a good treatment and that "the old Andy" was returning. In spite of my training as a psychiatrist, I struggled to make sense of what had happened during this two-year period of fluctuating hypomania, to identify how much was the illness and how much responsibility Andy had for the particular ways the hypomania was manifest in his behavior, which had left me with a lot of residual feelings of anger and hurt from all the disruption his hypomanic behavior had caused. As he recovered, he talked about his illness and its effects with us. He apologized to me and the kids. It took me a long time to accept his apology. He talked with the kids about his family history of bipolar illness. He opened himself up more with other people. Even during this time, while things were getting better, I remained deeply on edge almost all of the time. Looking back on it, I think I was quite traumatized.

Even though I don't believe in keeping secrets and know how destructive it can be, I felt unable to talk about all that had happened in my personal life while I was at work. To do so, in my mind, would make me too exposed and even more vulnerable. Some elements of his illness were known or rumored in the palliative care community. I imagine that people spoke about it among themselves, but not with me, and the idea of being "talked about" made my stomach turn. I felt ashamed—by my inability to help Andy and prevent his troubles, by my own hurt and fragility. We were so interconnected, in our own eyes and in those of others, that we were perceived as a unit, which made me feel somehow ashamed. I experienced a sense of isolation and felt people in my professional community had withdrawn from me. As I look back on it, I think that I also played a part in creating distance between myself and my colleagues. I did not ask for help at work and did not feel that I received it, although I suspect people may have been trying to help in ways that I simply could not see. Or perhaps I conveyed that I was OK or that it was not OK to reach out. I don't know.

Over time, life settled down. We worked hard to recover ourselves and our relationship. I was able to focus better on my work and learned how to be a department chair under less duress. My sense of competence and confidence in myself began to return. I had new and exciting projects and started to develop the Serious Illness Care Program. Andy and I started to have fun again. We had several marvelous trips to the UK, visiting Josh at Cambridge and then going to London or Paris for theater and museums, wonderful dinners, and lovely time together. But I still found myself constantly braced for Andy's hypomania to return or for his behavior to suddenly change.

Three years after Andy's hypomania episode began, just as life was beginning to smooth out, I became sick with gastrointestinal symptoms that were diagnosed as ulcerative colitis, a disease my mother had also had. I was sick for three years from the disease and also from the miserable, toxic, and ineffective drugs I tried. I was always exhausted, and several times became so sick that I required hospitalization. I remember lying on the floor in my office, vomiting into my wastebasket, and having to ask a colleague to help me get to the emergency room. I hated the disease. I hated what it did to me. I hated how it made me feel, and I hated feeling so vulnerable. I was struck by my comfort in caring for vulnerable people and my discomfort with my own vulnerability.

I grieved for my good health and tried to adjust to life with a chronic illness while still dealing with my unresolved feelings about Andy's hypomania. I wondered how all the stress I had experienced had impacted my immune system and how it might have contributed to the emergence of the ulcerative colitis. I was scared the whole time that we would not be able to get my symptoms under control. Partly because of my own stigmatization of the disease, I felt unsafe sharing information about my illness, although a few people knew that I was sick.

Andy was in much better shape, and I was lucky that he could finally support me. The kids and my closest friends were amazing, and therapy helped. We traveled and had good times in spite of my ongoing symptoms, which I was able to manage in a way so that most people around me were, I think, unaware of what I was dealing with. We went to Singapore to run a two-week faculty training program and spent a week at a lovely resort in Indonesia. We helped Josh move into a new apartment in New Haven as he started his life as a faculty member at Yale. We visited Gabe in California and spent time hiking and hanging out with close friends and our families.

I realize now how much the pressure I felt to be "a leader" affected me. I felt I had to be strong and that I could not allow people to see me as anything other than completely capable. I was creating a new department, in a new field, in a notoriously tough institution. It was a challenging role, even under the best of circumstances. And it felt like a very public role. I was supposed to be a change agent, but many well-meaning and established physicians did not think change was needed in the way we cared for patients with serious illnesses like cancer. I could see change, over the fifteen years I had been there, but it was slow, laborious, and stressful. I used to tell people "if you are not meeting resistance, you are not really doing change," but working against resistance was hard. For example, when I first arrived, I was called into the office of one of the executives who was upset that a poster about a teaching session about bereavement had been posted on a bulletin board that might be seen by patients. I was required to remove the poster; by the time I left, we did outreach to every bereaved family whose loved one had died and had received care at our institution, and we regularly posted notices about bereavement teaching, support groups, etc. throughout the institution.

Almost every innovation we introduced—from the palliative care clinical program, to a requirement that all patients complete a healthcare proxy early in their care trajectory, to communication training programs—elicited pushback. Although I had phenomenal support from institutional leadership, and many of the clinicians welcomed us with gratitude and appreciation, there was outright hostility to palliative care in some areas. Some clinicians believed strongly that they knew how to care for their own patients' palliative care needs and that we did not add anything. Others saw us as undermining their efforts to cure their patients, or worried we would upset their patients, or felt like we were a symbol of their inadequacy. Being an agent of change is deeply lonely. Looking back, I realize how unsafe I felt in that environment, particularly in the early years, as our department was being established. I always felt like an outsider. In the past, I had, in some ways, felt empowered and freed by being an "outsider" and being able to hew to my own goals and values and change agenda. But here, I felt that being too much of an outsider could compromise my effectiveness in making change as we slowly and carefully eked out every small innovation, titrating them to what was acceptable to our colleagues without too much tension and conflict. Although these perceptions abated somewhat over time, they were a constant feature of my experience.

As our department grew, I became less lonely in one way as we recruited and nurtured spectacular clinicians of many disciplines. I was not the only one speaking out about the importance of palliative care. My departmental colleagues felt like "my people" and were a great source of strength and support, even if most of it was indirect. I learned one of the hard lessons of leadership—that one can't really be "friends" with the people one is responsible for leading. I had lots of friendly relationships in my department, but did not feel that I could confide in my colleagues. This contributed to my sense of loneliness at work, as did being the first female department chair in my institution.

Although I was comfortable sharing my vulnerability in teaching settings, because I saw that it often facilitated more open and fruitful learning experiences and gave others permission to be more open, I only saw negatives in sharing my personal issues at work. Unconsciously, my perception of "leadership" was influenced by what I saw and felt around me, which was rather impersonal, business-like, and cool. I couldn't really do that, but I could not figure out a comfortable way to be a leader and also be myself.

People also saw me through their own emotional needs and histories. My job was to take care of the faculty and staff and to help them get what they needed to do their jobs well. I often felt overwhelmed by their wants and needs—someone didn't like her office, a talented faculty member needed some resources to do an important project, this person was having trouble in her job but had difficulty hearing feedback—it was incessant. Although in many ways I enjoyed the problem-solving components of learning how to build new programs to benefit patients and their families, as well as the interpersonal problem-solving of supporting a mentee who was trying to create her own path in our system, it was also exhausting. I worried about my effectiveness, about my illness, and about how Andy's troubles affected peoples'

views of me. Did they think less of me? How much more would I be marginalized if they knew I was chronically ill? I really did not want to be a subject of
gossip, and I knew it was happening.

One experience reinforced how dangerous it was to exhibit weakness, perceived or otherwise. I returned from medical leave and one of my faculty
members told me that she and other faculty from my department had been
invited to a secret meeting by another chair to try to coax them to leave our
department, and join his. This ugly power grab was quelled by institutional
leaders but reinforced my feeling that it was unsafe to share anything about
my personal situation at work.

I would regularly leave my office to receive treatment at the infusion center
of my own hospital in the middle of my workday, but I never told anyone,
apart from my beloved assistant, Cheryl, where I was going. I blamed myself for the difficulties in controlling my disease. I understand now the enormous gap between what was going on within me and how I was trying to
present myself in the outside world. On the one hand, trying to be composed,
keeping myself focused on work, solving problems, engaging with ideas, and
experiencing a sense of competence and productivity helped still the anxiety
I felt about my health and my personal life but also, at the same time, divided
my perception of my sense of self. There was so much disconnect, as if I were
living two lives at once.

At the same time, there were many exciting and engaging opportunities,
and I felt energized to take some risks professionally. In spite of my health
issues, I threw myself fully into developing the Serious Illness Care Program,
working with an incredible team and envisioning how this program could
have a broad impact on improving care for people with serious illness. Again,
work felt stabilizing and generative and heartening at a time when I needed
affirmation.

Then, in 2013, two years after my diagnosis, Andy was diagnosed with an
aggressive, "double-hit" lymphoma (how do they come up with a name like
this?). As difficult as it was, we both felt that "we knew how to do this" and
that our combined seventy years of palliative care involvement helped us
know what we were in for and how we might cope. Andy's mental health issues had made it necessary for both of us to do a lot of work on ourselves and
learn how to love each other better and more resiliently despite life's stressors.

In some ways, Andy's mental health crisis meant we were even more
closely connected in confronting his illness, which made everything easier.
Our kids wanted to be fully involved, and we spoke openly with them, and

we gathered close with the people we loved. We did not hesitate to call on friends, and they responded well to our openness. We found good doctors, talked with them about what mattered to us, evaluated options, and imagined the future. We were given clear information about the prognosis and a good understanding of the numbers, which framed our thinking. There was, according to the doctors, a small but meaningful (25–40%?) chance of a cure with aggressive treatment. We realized that we would have to be in some "middle space" of not knowing how things would turn out, living our lives with an awareness of both the good and bad outcomes in mind. We talked about what would be best for me to do about work if Andy lived and what would be best if he died. We were both afraid that if he died and I had left my work, I would be alone and without a structure for my life. We decided to see how it worked for me to stay in my job, delegate more, try to work more from home, step away from national activities, and get more help at home. It seemed like a reasonable compromise. We tried to support our kids in living their lives but also recognized how important it was to them to be part of this experience with us and how comforting it was for all of us to be together. Somehow, in spite of Gabe living on the West Coast and Josh living a few hours away, it felt like they were right there with us, every step of the way. Sometimes I worry that we leaned too much on them during that time.

Andy chose to undergo six months of aggressive chemotherapy, followed by radiation therapy, and he bore it stoically. We talked a lot about the future, with and without him. We "pre-enjoyed" events that had not happened yet, imagining what they might be like and how we would feel. We cried. We hoped. We tried to live. Andy spent most of the summer on our purple couch in the living room, often huddled under a blanket. He slept and read, and our close friends visited. When he felt good, we went to concerts or on walks. The kids came and went. With all of this, we were all still working on the hard things that had happened in our family. It was hard to process the unresolved issues from the past when Andy was so sick and vulnerable.

I continued to have symptoms, but dealing with Andy's illness and trying to work made it difficult to focus on myself. He had little energy, and read or visited with friends while I was at work. My most vivid memory of that time was of finishing the two-week faculty development course Andy and I had always taught together—an exhausting, all-in emotional experience—and feeling particularly bereft and fragile trying to run the course without him, dealing with my own feelings, and trying to support our learners. I felt comfortable and confident doing the teaching, but the emptiness and aloneness while running the course were intense. When we flew to Puerto Rico together at the end of the course to celebrate the end of his chemotherapy, we both collapsed in exhaustion. I remember how nurturing the lovely hotel felt in the midst of so much caretaking of everyone else—I had no responsibilities, the warm breeze flowed over us wherever we were, and we were surrounded by gorgeousness. It was a peaceful respite in a really bleak time.

We returned, and Andy underwent his radiation treatment. He was exhausted and depressed, and I took care of him. Even when professional colleagues from around the country organized a gathering in Andy's honor to lift his spirits and express appreciation and respect, Andy could not believe that they had come to support him, and us. I was getting sicker, having unremitting symptoms, and did not have further treatment options besides surgery. We kept trying to live as normal a life as we could, but it couldn't be normal, and I saw how the incredible stress of trying to do this and worrying and taking care of Andy must have exacerbated my illness. Work was a blur, even as it steadied me and reminded me of my strengths. And, if things went badly for Andy, it gave me a place to be in the world. Unconsciously, I think I was terrified of losing that lifeline, that crucial part of my identity.

As my symptoms got worse, it was clear that I had to have a colectomy. I was distraught about the surgery, but wanted to get it done. I told people I was having surgery, but was not specific with many people about what kind it was. One of my colleagues graciously stepped in as Acting Chair while I was away. When I went to surgery, Andy was still recovering from his radiation and tried to help, but he was also immobilized by depression and exhaustion. The kids were magnificent, calling every night, visiting when they could, but we didn't want them to have to be so heroic.

Once I had the surgery, I was quite sick afterward for a month or so as my body got used to the new internal arrangements. Andy was having trouble taking care of me, and his depression dulled his capacity to see and address, for example, an episode of severe dehydration that made me unable to get out of bed. Over the phone, a friend stepped in and assertively told me I needed to go to the hospital, where I stayed for several days. It was terrifying, but clarifying, to realize that my executive functions, and Andy's, were so bad that we couldn't recognize how sick I was and do what was needed.

I didn't want the kids to leave their lives to take care of me, and I asked my best friend, Mary, to come from California. We have been there for each other for everything—her parents' divorce, her brother's death, our mothers' deaths, the trials of motherhood, her divorce, and Andy's mental health crisis.

Her arrival in the house was like sunlight and hope and calm and competence and love, all bundled into one wonderful human being. I listened to her when she said I was strong and would get through this. I trusted her judgment. She was upbeat and was able to see what I needed before I knew I needed it. She reminded me to drink water; she cooked meals, brought me Popsicles, and joked around with Andy. And we talked. All of a sudden, things felt safe and under control at home. Andy's spirits improved. I adapted, with many glitches, as my body adjusted to a new reality. We spent time at our house in the Berkshires that summer, which had always been a peaceful refuge for us, where I rode my bicycle and regained confidence in my physical self. Andy was in remission, and we were hopeful. Life seemed more normal. I felt healthy for the first time in several years.

A few months later, taking advantage of Andy's remission, Gabe went to Paris for a month to learn some new lab techniques. I went to visit him, and Josh and Andy went to New York for a long weekend of opera, museums, good food, and hanging out. At the opera with Josh, Andy found a lump on his leg and realized his cancer was back. A few days later he picked me up at the airport and we drove directly to a conference in Vermont where we were both scheduled to give talks. After we had both finished giving our presentations, we returned to our hotel room and he told me that the cancer was back. It was beyond devastating—even though we had known this was a strong possibility all along, it felt like the bottom of the world had dropped out. I felt terrible that Andy had been holding this knowledge for twenty-four hours without telling me. We lay on the bed and held each other. We drove home from Vermont weeping. It was raining, and I was crying, and Vermont was explosive with fall color; the vibrant red and orange and yellow felt like an insult. We talked about how to tell the kids. Even though we had not spoken yet with the doctors, we both understood that Andy would probably die from the disease. We were heartsick and full of dread.

The doctors recommended a "tandem transplant," which involved two back-to-back stem-cell transplants; we were told this offered a 15–25% chance of long-term remission/cure. It was not obvious to Andy (or me) that he should go through another round of treatment. The decision felt impossibly heavy. Andy and I had both taken care of patients undergoing stem-cell transplant and had seen up close the difficult realities of this treatment— pain, terrible infections, graft versus host disease, death. And we had also seen people, including a good friend, be cured. I think we talked about everything that we were thinking, even though it was hard. We thought about lost time now versus potential time later if he went for this rigorous form of treatment; we discussed his quality of life, with and without the transplants; we talked about accepting a palliative approach with near-certain death within a few months; and we talked about the disruption of the treatment to our sons' lives and my life, as well as our sense that we had more emotional work to do as a family to recover from Andy's hypomanic episode and which course would better allow that to unfold. We worried about how this experience would affect the life trajectories of our sons. All the choices felt impossible, and we knew that there was no "right" one.

Open conversations with Andy's wonderful oncologist made it clear that there were exit options, such as stopping anti-rejection medications if quality of life after the transplants was intolerable. This grim conversation gave Andy a sense of agency and control and also allowed him to make clear what quality of life he thought he would be willing to tolerate. He decided to go ahead with the transplants. He said to me privately that he would not have gone through with the transplants for himself but that he deeply wanted to be around for the kids and me. He felt the kids needed him and that the transplant was the best chance he had of being around for them. The kids and I felt it was entirely his decision, after we had all processed what the choices meant, and we were all committed.

When I learned that his lymphoma had returned, I stepped down from my role as Chair, and my colleague again took over as Acting Chair. In one way, leaving this job was a great loss, but in many others it was a tremendous relief—from the stress, the constant demands, and the pressure to be "on" all the time. I continued to be involved in my academic work but reduced my work commitments to meet the caretaking demands that Andy's two transplants would create. In some ways, it felt even more urgent not to give everything up because it was now much more likely Andy would die. There is a lot of downtime when someone is very ill and having something that I cared about to occupy my mind helped. But work felt very secondary. I went to occasional meetings. I did conference calls from the waiting room while Andy was on the transplant unit. I remember the time of his transplants as like being in a bubble with him, our kids, and the clinical team. Friends dropped off meals, did some driving, and talked for hours on the phone when I was feeling despondent. Our life felt like it orbited entirely around Andy's illness.

Andy was miserable, both in the hospital and at home. We had to be super careful about cleaning everything he touched to avoid infection while his immune system was recovering. He was not allowed to eat food that was not prepared at home, could not eat uncooked vegetables and many fruits, and had to avoid certain cheeses. Preparing meals and keeping the house clean felt a bit like walking through landmines, as there were so many ways that he could get an infection. He could not leave the house except to sit outside or go to the cancer center, friends could not visit at first, and then only with face masks. There were many unexpected visits to the doctor and the emergency department.

Andy cherished the time with Josh and Gabe. When they came, they would swoop into the house and cook and fix whatever technology we had disrupted, and we would sit around together in different configurations. I remember there were a lot of movies. We talked about how Andy was doing, how we were each managing, and a lot of ordinary things. There was joking around, which had always been a feature of our family life. There was a sorrowful peace in the house when we were all there. The presence of the kids always lifted me up, and I remember a sense of unbearable loss every time they would leave.

This continued for about seven months, mostly in Cambridge and, during the summer, at our house in the Berkshires. In August, because of side effects and worsening lab values, some of Andy's anti-rejection medications were reduced, and he started to feel better. We rejoiced. I went to California to watch Gabe defend his dissertation at Stanford. Josh came to stay with Andy while I was gone. Andy and Josh watched the streamed version of Gabe's thesis defense from Cambridge, cheering him on. Josh and Andy had some important time together. Gabe and I were able to celebrate his PhD; take some short, spectacular hikes into the high Sierras; and begin his road trip from California back to Boston, where he was moving for his post-doc. Josh left soon after I returned from California to start his sabbatical year in Washington, DC. Andy's sense of well-being returned during this time, and, for the first time on the day Gabe was arriving from California, Andy said he could envision this whole terrible experience being behind him. We fantasized about a trip to Hawaii, all of us together.

The next night, for the first time in eight months, Andy and Gabe and I went out to dinner to celebrate Andy's seventieth birthday, which seemed like a momentous landmark in what looked like might be at least a tentative recovery. We sat outside on the terrace of a lovely country inn, about twenty-five minutes from our house, because Andy was not allowed to sit inside and risk infection. The three of us had a warm, tender, silly, and touching evening with two close friends. Andy ate roast duck, his favorite dish. There was a lot of joking, he toasted all of us individually and thanked us for helping him get to this point. We celebrated Gabe's arrival from California. I don't remember much of the conversation, only that Andy seemed to have recovered his usual playful spirit that I loved. It was an exquisite evening. For the first time since the transplants, Andy felt well enough to drive us all home from dinner.

But then, the next day, Andy woke up feeling terrible. He could not get out of bed. He was so sick he couldn't say good-bye to our beloved friends who were returning to Chicago that day. We were very scared. He had had some episodes like this during the post-transplant period, but this was different. We worried about food poisoning. Or worse. I drove him into Boston, a sense of dread weighing me down.

The team was unsure what was going on. Andy developed terrible abdominal pain and was hospitalized, still without a diagnosis. Josh flew back to Boston so all four of us were together. Andy was very confused and scared and could not make decisions for himself. After talking with the kids, I directed the doctors to treat him aggressively, as Andy had said he would want, in the hope that this acute episode was reversible. He was transferred to the ICU to be on a ventilator so that he could be sedated comfortably and have a biopsy to see if the process was treatable. Five days after his admission, in a strange twist, my gastroenterologist, who was the "attending" doctor in the ICU, came to tell us the results of Andy's biopsy. I could not figure out why he was there and why he looked so upset when he saw me. The biopsy showed that Andy had a complication of the transplant—severe graft versus host syndrome, in which the transplanted cells attack the person's own cells, causing intense inflammation and pain. The extent of the new process, as well as the fact that it was affecting his kidneys, brain, and other organs, indicated that Andy was extremely unlikely to survive. Josh and Gabe and I made the decision together to withdraw life-sustaining treatments. The frenetic rush and commotion of his medical management gave way to a quieter and slower process of saying good-bye. Over the next twenty-four hours, Andy's brother and cousin and friends came to visit. Andy died gently in the ICU, with us around him and Bach playing in the background. We were full of sorrow, and we were also at peace.

I thought that I knew how to grieve. I saw grief as pure and even kind of beautiful because of how it revolved around love and connection. It was hard, but it did not undermine my fundamental sense of self. I had control over myself, and I could create my own way through the process, one that made sense to me and offered comfort. I had grieved for my mother when I was in my twenties and for my father in my fifties. I had been with many patients over the years as they grieved loved ones.

In spite of my intellectual sense of preparation and incredible support from Josh and Gabe, the rest of my family, my work community, and my friends, I felt sad, lost, alone, vulnerable, and unprotected. My kids and I had a tremendous sense of solidarity. We were each going through our own versions of sorrow, alone and together. The closeness that I felt with them when Andy was sick continued after his death. We were bereft and fragile, but emotionally connected. Although Josh returned to his sabbatical home in Washington, DC, a week or so after Andy died, our "threeness" was sustaining during that time.

Gabe had moved into our house while getting settled in Boston. We tried to focus on his goals before Andy got sick and on helping him find a place to live. He bought a condo nearby. He had always planned to get a dog when he finished his PhD. We debated whether this was a terrible time or the best possible time to get a puppy. And so, five weeks after Andy's death, we brought home a sweet pup from the shelter. Argos brought love, ridiculousness, and joy into our sad household, where our dog, Waldo had been in deep mourning with us for Andy. Many of the grief books advise the bereaved not to make any major life changes in the year after a loss; both Gabe and I felt that bringing this new, vulnerable, wild, scared, Georgia "rainbow dog" into our home was an affirmation that life goes on. The moments of joy and silliness were exquisite in the middle of so much sorrow.

After Gabe moved into his new condo with Argos, I began to focus on my own feelings. I wasn't surprised when I experienced a resurgence of hurt and anger related to Andy's hypomanic behavior; I was especially angry because it felt like we had lost those years together as a couple and as a family. I questioned, again, my own actions during that time. I loved and supported him through all of his difficulties, even though I believed that I had paid a significant price with my own emotional and physical health. I experienced a deep sense of gratitude that he had had time to accept and understand his illness, been able to apologize for and acknowledge how it had affected him, and make amends with me and with the kids for its effects on us.

I also began preparing for a life alone. I told myself that I would "just say yes" to every invitation and weird opportunity that came my way. I tried a bunch of new things. I went to a restaurant bar and had dinner for the first time by myself when I was on a work trip. I asked my son, Josh, how to negotiate this. He suggested I chat with the bartender, so, when I was in London for work, I went to a terrific restaurant where I ordered a nice dinner and a glass of good wine. I felt awkward but determined. I confessed to the bartender that I had never done this before, and he laughed at me and poured me a second glass of wine. I watched people in the mirror at the back of the bar and enjoyed the sociability. I considered it a success. I went to some very mediocre and one terrible poetry reading. I spent three weeks with my friend, Mary, on the Northern California coast, fostering a basket of abandoned puppies.

During this time, I had an urgent drive to "do it now." I was processing a lot of hard feelings and feeling bereft and intensely aware of the unpredictability and tragedy of life. I was still hurting and vulnerable from going through Andy's hypomanic episode. I didn't want to delay things that I had always said I wanted to do. Eight months after Andy died, I decided to rebuild our summer house in Western Massachusetts that had been, for twenty years, a place of peace and togetherness for our family and with our dear friends who had built a house next door. Andy and I had talked about someday doing a renovation, but it was never the right time. I had always wanted to build a house—my mother and I used to design houses on paper for various locations that we discovered in the Sierras in California. I wanted to do something that was different from the old house but connected to our past, something that would make me happy and be a place where I could spend time with my two sons, and, I hoped, eventually their families. So, after exploring lots of options, I knocked down our old house and built a new house on the original foundation, with the same basement stairs we had in the old house. It was a scary, wonderful, hopeful experience, and the process, as well as the finished house, gives me great joy. In some ways I saw it as something I was doing to memorialize Andy—the house represented our intact family, our love for the Berkshires, the memories, and the future. When the house was finished, I knew that Andy would have loved it.

The second most surprising thing about my life in the time after Andy died was the intense and painful sense of vulnerability I had in my work environment. I can't really be sure how much was my state of mind and how much was a change in the way I was treated. I felt incredibly fragile—as if I had no skin between me and the world. So things that happened at work hurt. A lot. Because Andy and I had worked closely together, we had always had a sense of mutual protection and support. I didn't have that any more.

Around the time of Andy's death, after a search that began when I left my position the previous year, a new chair started in my old role. I refocused on my work on the Serious Illness Care Program at a separate lab in order to give the new chair space to lead the department, although I hoped to continue in some small role in the department. I thought that by relocating most of my work outside my old department, I could continue to make meaningful contributions, collaborate with terrific people, and be out of the way of the new chair. I hoped this plan could offer me a gradual and graceful path toward retirement over multiple years, one that might allow me to be a support to the new chair and have some small role in the department.

It didn't turn out that way. After I returned to work following Andy's death, I felt a real emotional chill in my work settings. I was perplexed by the change in what I experienced. I felt unwelcome at the lab and in my old department.

At the lab, I realized there had been some significant administrative changes that left me feeling I had no voice about how the team that I had founded and built would do our Serious Illness Care Program work. After a long track record in multiple leadership roles and many wonderful experiences mentoring young faculty and staff, I found it untenable to be told that I could not lead my own team the way I wanted to lead it. I was shocked and upset to find myself excluded from conversations about the program. I expressed my concerns and did not feel listened to. I felt completely powerless, like I had become invisible.

In my old department, it was made clear to me that there was no place for me to be part of this new phase of its development, except through seeing patients. Again, I was hurt and angry. After appealing to my old boss, I was "allowed" to go back to teaching what had been a successful seminar for fellows and faculty that I had run off and on for many years. I loved the teaching and was happy to have this small connection to my old department.

I initially attributed what was happening to my grief and worried that I was doing something to elicit these behaviors or that I was misperceiving them. I thought that perhaps people were reacting to the fact that I had been away from work for a great deal of the prior year and that others had taken on new roles and developed new ways of doing things. I wondered if people really didn't like or want to work with me, but I could not reconcile that with my own experiences and the feedback that I had received. I wondered if there was something scary about the way I represented a reminder to people about potential loss. I thought back on the experience during my medical leave, when a colleague tried to take over part of my department, and wondered whether woundedness somehow was threatening and elicited aggression. In truth, I felt attacked and undermined, particularly by several colleagues whom I had supported earlier in their careers and whom I had thought were friends. I wondered whether they needed to destroy me, or vanquish me, in order to feel their own strength. It was hard to imagine that anyone could think I was threatening or needed to be vanquished because I felt so fragile, lost, and diminished in my grief. It was unspeakably painful.

And so, in this unexpected way, I was mired in a new kind of unhappiness. I took care of my patients. I tried to take care of the faculty I was responsible for. I tried to keep growing the Serious Illness Care Program. I believed in it, and I cared deeply about the faculty.

While still in the midst of dealing with all of this, a regular screening MRI that I get annually because of a strong family history of pancreatic cancer showed a pancreatic mass, which was thought to likely be pancreatic cancer. Three years after the death of their father, I had to prepare my kids for what we were told was an overwhelming likelihood that I had pancreatic cancer. After a period of testing and biopsies, and multiple opinions from experts, I had a Whipple procedure to remove and biopsy my pancreas. It is a complex surgery. I remembered that, when I was in medical school, people spoke about "a Whipple" in hushed, horrified voices, and that image of the surgery hovered in my mind.

The Whipple showed that I had autoimmune pancreatitis. They removed it. I was fine. Except for the recovery. Having a second autoimmune disorder made me worry about the level of stress I had been under at work and what role it played in my health. While I was recovering from the surgery, I decided it would be better for me to disconnect from my role with the Serious Illness Care Program. I didn't think I could or should continue to work in such a stressful and toxic environment. I found other projects I wanted to pursue. I began teaching a Freshman Seminar at Harvard College; I continued to see a small number of patients; I started taking Italian classes; I took several printmaking courses; I worked on several academic projects.

Leaving then and in that way was not what I wanted, and I felt an enormous sense of sadness and loss. I felt I still had a lot to contribute, but I didn't want to struggle so hard and I didn't want to start up in a new institution or take on a new and stressful job. It was a terrible and humiliating way to end my career, which had been, up until this period, marked by widely recognized good work. But given the circumstances, and especially my health issues and the unhappiness my work situation was causing me, it felt like the best decision I could make, but there was a feeling of defeat in not having a better option.

In retrospect, I would have wished my career to have ended at the time I stepped down as chair, when Andy had become sick again, when I felt loved and respected at work. I feel emotionally brutalized and profoundly perplexed by the experiences I had in these last years at work. I have always thought of myself as a perceptive and empathic person, and I am troubled by the concern about what in myself I am not seeing. Why did this happen?

Over time, as I began to recover some from my grief and global vulnerability, I recognized that an additional factor was at play. As I realized that the people who were having a problem with me were men, it led me to think about the role of sexism in my story. As a strong-minded, direct, successful, and perceptive woman, I was likely seen as a threat. But during this time, my experience was of crying secretively in the bathroom, sometimes in grief, sometimes in frustration and hurt at what I was experiencing at work. I certainly did not perceive myself as a threat to anyone. I was told by one of the men that I was not "likable" and by another that my leadership style was too "strong." Although I intellectually could see that these comments were tropes that many men applied to women leaders, I still was afraid that they were correct and that I had failed. I could not take in the information that countered that external narrative, and I felt damaged, diminished, and betrayed by what I experienced as mistreatment and disrespect from men with whom I thought I had good relationships. I heard similar stories from other women. It took me a long time, but I felt I had to address the sexism issues directly with the individuals involved, both for my own self-respect but, most importantly, because I heard about and saw the same behavior happening to others. I realized that I was less vulnerable than I felt, and I recognized my responsibility, as a senior woman, to name what I realized was happening for the younger women who were more vulnerable than I was. After I did this, my anger fell away quite a bit, and I felt a sense of relief and restored self-esteem to have spoken up, even though I did not see anything change.

I have also reflected on the privilege of power that I had for twenty years and how a title and leadership role can insulate one from the harshness of medical culture and competition. I believe that some of the experiences I had after Andy's death were those of returning to a life where I had lost my power; my strong reaction was to the shock of refamiliarizing myself with what lack of power feels like. The feelings of helplessness, being discounted, feeling devalued, and not feeling seen are deeply damaging. I hadn't felt that at work since I was a young faculty member, just starting out. When I did recognize the toxic effects of my own powerlessness, it began to change who I identify with and allowed me to see more clearly how power affects the powerful. Instead of identifying with "leadership," I could feel the pain of some of my junior colleagues, particularly those who felt excluded, particularly because of racism, sexism, or choosing a less traditional professional trajectory. I remember worrying, while I was a chair, about losing my empathy and how taking a fiduciary responsibility seriously and simultaneously acting empathically was sometimes impossible. I remember a situation in which I had to fire a long-term employee and how sure I was that what I was doing was best for the department because she was a disruptive presence who was holding others back, but I remember also feeling disturbed that I was not more upset by the idea of firing her, and I wondered at my capacity to do such a hurtful thing. My experiences in these recent years make me wonder what emotional deadening I didn't recognize when I had power.

Losing power, even voluntarily, is still a loss, and it changed my sense of where I fit in my work world. I liked feeling respected and sought after and admired, and I miss those reactions from others as my role has changed. As time has passed, and I have become more accepting of where I am in my life and more at peace with the decision I made to leave my institutional homes, I have discovered the joys of a slower, more flexible life, with time to explore new things; in this new reality, power seems like an illusion, with too high a cost, and I feel lucky to be free.

I had expected to be alone for the rest of my life. The most surprising thing in all that happened after Andy died was falling in love again, finding a good man and feeling our way into a future together.

Peter and I met socially for the first time a year after Andy died and months after his wife had also died. There were uncanny parallels in our lives. In addition to our shared recent experiences with losing beloved spouses, we were both on the medical school faculty at Harvard, lived in Cambridge, were red-diaper babies, subscribed to *The Nation* magazine, shared many political values, had summer houses—his on Martha's Vineyard and mine in the Berkshires—had lived in Europe as children, and had two grown children. As our relationship developed, I began to realize the ways that expecting to be alone was a way of protecting myself from my longings for connection and from the ways that relationships can be hard and heartbreaking.

Soon after Peter and I connected, my contractor, who had just begun working on my new Berkshire house, called me and told me he thought the bedroom was too small and that I should come out as soon as possible to the new house and take a look at the layout, which he had laid out in 2 × 4s on the floor. Thinking I would be alone, I had wanted to have a small bed-room to leave more of the house for common space. When Peter and I went out the next day to look, we realized that I had created a room suitable for a nun—tiny, barely enough room for a bed, no room for a bureau, and cer-tainly no room for a partner. I realized that I wanted space in my bedroom for a partner and for myself. Since all that existed was a floor, we were easily able to move the location of walls to create a bedroom in which two people could be comfortable.

Five years later, we are still finding our way together, both enjoying and struggling with coming together late in our lives and across big differences, but held together by love, humor, shared values, and the capacity to support and care for each other through the daily (and sometimes difficult) parts of our lives.

This story feels distant, but also intensely real, now six years after Andy's death. My sons continue to be a link to the past and the future, to all the joys and difficult times when we were originally a family of four with Andy. They are good men and are building meaningful lives. We have loved each other and hung together through all of this, although losing the "threeness" with them that was so powerful while Andy was ill and after his death was really hard for all of us. Andy is still very much present in my memory and especially when I am with Josh and Gabe. I cherish the ways that I see his strengths expressed in each of them.

For myself, what stays with me most powerfully from my experiences with the losses I describe here is a sense of my own strength, my deep love for the people who traveled so lovingly with me through this saga, and a mix of ac-ceptance, sorrow, and gratitude for my particular life. I have found my own way, with help, through the hard parts, tried to learn from them and grow as a person. As I look at myself now, I see myself growing and recognize that, as my work world has become small, my life has become big. The balance feels right.

Epilogue

I originally planned to co-edit this book with Matt. My decision to step away as co-editor came from a recognition of the uncertainties of this stage of life, perhaps amplified by such intense exposure to illness and death; an awareness of my own physical vulnerability and fragility, which call for my attention and effort to reduce stress and build strength and resilience; and the totally unexpected experience of having the opportunity to create a new life.

I feel a combination of guilt, sorrow, relief, and gratitude that I have had the opportunity to think and learn so deeply about loss from the colleagues who have opened themselves up in this book to share their own losses and have been moved by their honesty and courage. I appreciate Matt for his vision, and especially for his generosity in understanding my need to separate myself from this book project.

As I wrote this narrative and processed all the feelings that revisiting these events brought forth, I began to feel that I did not want to continue to live in the world of loss, even intellectually. I know loss will come again, but I have been living in and experiencing the world through a filter of loss for the past forty years, both through my work and, intensely, through the period I describe here. I want a break from this immersion in sorrow and heartache, to see what the world looks like without the constant exposure and preoccupation with all the hard things people experience through illness, death, and suffering.

About the Author

Susan D. Block, MD, is Professor of Psychiatry and Medicine at Harvard Medical School. Dr. Block has been a national leader in the development of the field of palliative medicine in the United States and, through her leadership of the Open Society Institute's Project on Death in America, trained and developed many of early leaders in the field. Subsequently, through her founding and leadership, the Department of Psychosocial Oncology and Palliative Care at Dana-Farber Cancer Institute and Brigham and Women's Hospital grew that interdisciplinary program into one of the largest and strongest palliative care programs in the country. With her husband and frequent collaborator, Andy Billings, she founded and co-directed the Harvard Medical School Center for Palliative Care, a national center of excellence in palliative care education, training thousands of clinicians from around the world in palliative care award-winning courses. In 2011, with Atul Gawande, she started and led the Serious Illness Care Program at Ariadne Labs, a joint center for healthcare innovation at Brigham and Women's Hospital and

Harvard School of Public Health, leading that program until 2017. She is the author of more than 200 publications. She has won numerous awards for education, research, and leadership. She currently leads a Freshman Seminar at Harvard University, Serious Illness, Death and Dying in the age of COVID-19; continues her palliative care teaching at Dana-Farber and Brigham and Women's Hospital; and works with a small number of patients.

11

"In Sickness and in Health, ' Til Death Do Us Part"

Marshall Forstein

> What we call the beginning is often the end
> And to make an end is to make a beginning
> The end is where we start from
>
> —T. S. Eliot[1]

We met, fell in love, and started a life together that lasted thirty-eight years before his illness and death tore us apart. Two gay men, one Black, one White, whose very existence was at that time seen as an anathema to much of society, alienated from the social rights and privileges of our heterosexual counterparts, creating a relationship against all odds beginning in 1980. We invented the rules of engagement, crossed chasms of institutionalized and internalized racism and homophobia, and put in place rituals to which we were told we were not entitled. Rebels with a cause. Confident, strident, terrified. Ours, now looking back, was an unexpected love.

Already together for twenty-four years, having adopted two children, built a family, a network of friends, and professional careers in the mental health field (me in psychiatry and him in psychology), we married legally, in 2004, in Massachusetts, and spoke those vows that foreshadow all relationships.

The problem was that his getting cancer and dying before me was not the plan ("man plans god laughs"). He came from a family of men with long lives, whereas my tribe's men died most often prematurely from heart disease. Thus, I expected and was prepared to die first and had all things prepared if that were to be the case: finances, paperwork, support for solo parenting adult children, the old house's unending needs, the appointments for the dogs' nails to be cut, food shopping, the changing of the multiple water filters hidden under cabinets (did he ever even know about their existence?), caulking the drafty old windows, and the endless futile attempt to clean the basement collection of decades of ours and others' forgotten treasures. In the fury to prepare for my own expected demise at some point, my obsessional traits found new ways to help ward off any other possible scenario.

Yet, in spite of this rational plan, I was angry that the universe did not conspire with me. Only now in retrospect can I admit that, had I gone first, he would not have been as prepared to manage the grief, and perhaps his life remaining, without me. Being the organized, obsessional one, the details of survivorship and the burden I now knew he would feel tempered the smoldering rage of abandonment. Even my sons were finally able to acknowledge that his passing first spared him the task of losing me and feeling unable to manage life by himself. Do all children have an unspoken anxiety about which parent will die first? Somehow, I felt a strange and unsettling comfort that if all that I could feel was grief I would wear it for both of us. Between the terror and the sadness, all was wrapped in a feeling of loss that coursed through me in spasms, pulses, and continuous pains through my body. The intensity of feeling vacillated between denial and overwhelming paralysis. What is the self-remaining, again alone after struggling so hard to cross that loneliness to know another? How does one learn to live alone after having had an accomplice in love?

In the Beginning

We met during my internship in 1980. Both recently out of relationships, we each had been committed to being alone for a time, and my schedule ensured that we would have limited time together to even imagine starting anew. I had never met anyone before with as many books as me (all read!) or vinyls with the enormous spectrum of music. We came from what on the surface may have looked like different worlds, one Black, one White, but it was clear that beneath our skin tones was much difference and similarity. Both endlessly opinionated. Boredom was not going to be a problem.

We met at a party for interns from two hospitals. Having gotten there a bit late after leaving work, I gobbled three brownies, the only food left on the table. Suddenly aware of the looks of my fellow partiers, I realized too late the true nature of the brownies and waited for the tsunami of intoxication. Sitting in the corner with friends, somehow finding myself playing with my hands in the air demonstrating the mime I had used with teens when teaching high school, he noticed me as he entered the party with his friends, and we exchanged looks across the room. I was smitten. We moved quickly from a first date to boyfriends, slowed only by my being on call every third night. For the first time, I was intoxicated as much by the mental and emotional as the physical connection, though I am at a loss to describe how they were different. Love followed crush rapidly.

Within a couple of months, it seemed clear to both of us that this relationship was getting increasingly serious. I think my visceral recognition that this man was going to change my life in unpredictable ways, and the defenses against that, came out one night when we were running around Lake Merritt in Oakland, near to where he was living. Although I cannot even recall what the subject of our first conflict was within months after meeting, I will never forget that I reacted to something he said that was both wonderful and terrifying in its implications. I stopped abruptly, and he followed suit, and I said without thinking, clearly a bit agitated, "You know, I didn't need to fall in love with a Black man!", to which he replied without missing a beat, with an unexpected smile, "Yes, you did." And he was right. Thus began our mutual journey through the complex issues of race, for us, our family, and friends.

Only together a few months, we decided to move to Boston for my residency, and he was more than eager to escape the family that pulled continuously from him.

The Beginning of the Middle

Three years after moving to Boston, we exchanged rings in the car stuck on Route 3 coming back from an intensely romantic weekend in Provincetown. What did the rings mean, we asked? How do we mark what others understand through rituals of thousands of years? We were connected and alive and something made sense without being fanciful. Perhaps it was the monotonous traffic crawl that accentuated the feelings that we were cocooned in the car, safe and feeling contained with the love we expressed in that most mundane of experiences. Moments of intense conversation punctuated by comfortable, reflective silences. Though I still talk to him, and I can feel and hear him, I can no longer look into his eyes, and I miss that dearly with an emptiness in my gut that seems to reach without ending until I am distracted back into the present.

After five years we adopted a baby and then five years later, a gay teenager who needed a home. We worked hard, made wonderful friends with neighbors and others, and tried to deal with the growing devastation of AIDS on our community, and to the illnesses and deaths of parents, uncles, aunts, etc. We were not strangers to pain, suffering, and death. Tears, grief, and loss were daily fare in the gay community, amid the growing awareness of same-sex relationships and the beginning of social acceptance. We were always acutely aware that, having met in 1980 in San Francisco at the beginning of the epidemic, had we not met when we did, we might not have lived out our life together, or at all. We learned all too early about the unceasing losses of friends and colleagues as we were just beginning our life together. At one point I realized that I was losing more friends than was my eighty-five-year-old grandmother. But with each of the losses that I continue to discover live within me, friends and colleagues who come to the fore of my mind unexpectedly in unpredictable moments, triggered by something unknown, I had him as a companion in grief. Carrying all that loss of our friends, family members, and colleagues was now mine alone. Although I knew this at some level, each memory of someone no longer here is a reminder that grief is the loneliest of journeys.

My residency started as the HIV epidemic was blossoming, and it propelled me into a career that others thought would be detrimental to my future due to the stigma associated with the epidemic. Nothing could have predicted how this choice brought me such a collection of friends and colleagues who have been such a major support for me through these past two difficult years. Becoming involved with death and dying, and then working in palliative care education and training, has been a gift and toughened my already thick New York City skin, and I think this has allowed me to work with others grieving while in the midst of my own grief. But I worried that my own grief impaired my listening to others in pain.

Parenting and developing our professional lives filled time and emotion. We felt the stark fortune in our lives as we watched illness and homophobia steal life from so many we loved. We were held by our families, our neighbors, and our lifelong friends from each of our pasts, bringing together a remarkable cacophony of voices and colors, interests and life experiences. Time, in retrospect, passed quickly, with our sons growing into men, and, suddenly, we were the "older generation."

Together we twice weathered the trials of our sons' adolescence. We learned, or rather, were instructed by the boys, how to be the parents they needed. My father, with whom my husband had grown very close, reminded us in a phrase that "if you leave your kids alone, they'll bring you up right." He didn't mean it the way it sounds. In fact, he was an ever-present father, but he understood that every child has to be him- or herself, not a projection of our own failed attempts or unmet expectations. That advice was also about the two of us loving the person for who he was, not who we wanted him to be. This became so very difficult for me to see and be OK with, with my husband dealing with his cancer on his terms when I wanted so intensely to take care of it all.

We had "practice" with the dying of our friends and our dogs, who never seem to outlive us. We carried each other through the deaths of our parents, nurtured our griefs, and recognized that we were the next generation to be called to death and that we were now the ones who stood before our sons having to face mortality. And when his diagnosis was made and we quickly came to understand that we would lose to this cancer, not today, but in some foreshortened time, we fought to keep the fear of death and detachment at bay until we could no longer. We lived the first four years of his cancer as though it was a nuisance. I fought to keep my medical knowledge at bay, titrating how much research and information I could tolerate while trying to make sure he was getting the best treatment. We continued with our lives, working, playing when we could, punctuated with the unending trips to doctors and labs, imaging, and occasionally an emergency room. We planned, and then had to put off, some travel that took us farther than a weekend away.

Soon after his diagnosis, our younger son, who had broken up with his long-time girlfriend, moved back into the house with the thought of re-turning to school and starting up his artwork and music with a seriousness that was stunning to both of us. His working at home in a studio he built made him available to be a primary caretaker and, most importantly, companion, once the illness kept my husband at home more and more. We bonded even more with the recognition that the entire family and close friends shared the experience of his cancer. The small losses were almost imperceptible in the moment, yet shocking when we stopped to realize where we were com-pared to a year before. Almost every aspect of life became infiltrated with the impact of these losses. As was my style, as his illness progressed, I accom-modated, always trying to find the most positive perspective, harboring the anger at his illness and the growing insight into how much more was placed on me to carry. Increasingly, I felt the creeping into our lives of the tension between being a couple and the awareness of the inevitability of being alone.

I was more comfortable with the prospect of being alone as I had been alone several times in my life thus far, but I realized that loneliness is more painful when it is felt within the relationship, though I dared not allow feeling angry at him for getting sick. I had worked with couples, both dying of AIDS, who had conveyed a sense of comfort in them going through this together until the final stages when one left the other and the surviving one experienced often the terror of suddenly realizing he would die alone. I was mortified at my selfish feeling of relief that I was not the one dying and yet guilty as well.

Then there was sex, or rather, there wasn't. Not long after he was diagnosed with the prostate cancer, he began treatment using an anti-androgen intended to stop the growth of the cancer. Lupron, twisted in my imagination into something reminding me of the Latin word for wolf, *lupus*, further occupying mind space with the metaphor "wolf in sheep's clothing" when in fact what the medication did was make my husband the virile wolf into a tender, vulnerable lamb, robbing him of the body that we both loved. We struggled. Me toward him mostly at first, rebuffed by his own shame about his body. We found safe spaces to hold each other, silently most of the time, whispering our love that had nothing to do with sex and everything to do with our sexuality. I don't quite remember when in the five years of his illness he told me he was fine with me seeking pleasure elsewhere: "I know what you need, and I can't give it to you." I told him after three decades I was not going anywhere. In the private moments, each loss was met with tears of unending sadness and inevitability. This "thing" we had fashioned together began to fray at the edges as he pulled more into himself, leaving me to wonder: Who was I to become? The slow loss of him as husband, lover, friend, co-parent, intellectual partner, and caretaker was suffered alone.

The illness progressed. I cannot remember when he just stopped driving, going out on his own, holding court at home with friends when he would let them come keep company, especially while I was at work. Our evenings were filled with making meals, encouraging him to stay hydrated, and watching British comedies and dramas. Old friends would call, but he was increasingly isolating and more depressed, something he had suffered with episodically throughout his life. Treatments became more intense, and then, suddenly, we were told that the treatment was not working and that there was nothing new to offer chemotherapeutically. I kept searching the medical literature obsessively, sure there was something magical we had missed. Eventually, I had to be satisfied that his treatment team was in fact on top of the newest, even experimental treatments. Being a physician, I struggled with the feeling of being out of control, of being helpless to turn this around. I raged at the difference between the betrayal of the body and being hurt by an outside force, an accident, a hate crime, a slip and crack of the head. We are not taught, but have to learn and intuit, about the humility that being a physician requires when we go up against a deranged cell, a mutated piece of the self. It was at this point, I now realized, I began to grieve, and I had to find spaces to do so. Running in the park with the dogs gave me time to cry and pull myself back together before returning to the house. Did he know of my unspoken terror that I would lose him?

The Ending

Forgetting is not a choice. There are moments frozen in mind that one would hope to forget. Memories contain all we wish to hold onto and much we would will ourselves to forget. About 9 P.M. one night, as I was upstairs cleaning up, he texted me from downstairs as he found it hard to yell by this time such that I could hear him. <<I'm bleeding>> was all it said. I ran downstairs to find him holding a towel between his legs, a slow trickle of bright red blood visible when I moved the towel. I told my son that I was taking him to the emergency room and would call him once we knew what was happening. I tried to be calm and assuring, while instantly fearing that we were at some watershed. I had just enough medical knowledge to worry about all sorts of things that would forever change our lives. My body chilled as though I had slipped into icy waters, struggling to keep afloat while trying to find the shore.

Hours in the ER, finally scanned and comfortable while they waited to admit him. My heart was heavy, knowing that he was scared and that I was helpless to fix what was happening. Somewhere in the back of my mind I remember thinking, "too soon, not yet, not ready," as though one could ever be ready.

Over the next ten days, I stayed almost continuously in the hospital as they struggled to stop the slow and steady bleeding in his bladder. Transfusions, decisions about what to try next, and a slow recognition day after day and nights I spent in the hospital that he might never come home. I called and emailed our families and friends about the acute situation and the fear that he would never leave the hospital, and people showed up, relieved me for an hour or two so I could go home, change clothes, shower, and regroup. His mental state actually seemed to calm once we knew that we were near the end. I knew he was exhausted and was more worried about me than him-self. We spent hours talking about everything, and he said he was ready. We gathered one afternoon with friends and family who could make the trek and celebrated his seventy-first birthday in the hospital. He extracted promises from me about what I would do after he was gone, the first time he stated out loud that he was aware he was dying. We talked about all the things he wanted for me, the boys, our home, and how I was to live the rest of my life. Those moments of such brutal openness, and honesty, were at once monuments to an exquisite feeling of love and impending doom. I can hold those moments in my mind's eye as though suspended in time when I need to "feel" him with me.

Profoundly sad, I thought my tortured heart would break into pieces. I think I was more terrified than he was. We talked, held each other as if time had stopped, though I could feel he was trying to let go. I asked how he was feeling: "Scared?" He grabbed my hand harder and firm as if to reassure me, smiled, and said, "I'm curious." That was who he was throughout his life. Like a spear piercing my stomach, I knew this journey was his alone. Through my tears he made me smile and tell him that I would be all right and that I should tell the boys he loved them, and me, totally. I held his hand as he slipped gently into sleep. I slept in the chair next to him, fitfully, exhausted, and cold, and deeply alone.

Over the next twenty-four hours he slipped into a quiet, painless uncon-sciousness, until he was unarousable. Where are you? Where is all of us that we built? How do I let go?

When his breathing slowed, almost imperceptibly except to an as-tute person who had witnessed death before, I was caught between my horror at the reality of the moment *he* stopped breathing and the incessant observations of the body as I had witnessed so many times before through my training and working with dying patients in the early days of the AIDS epidemic. But this body had been warm moments before, and the mind plays tricks to see movement of the chest where there is none. Kindly, the nurse sitting with me through the last hour reached over and touched my arm and said, "He's gone." She told me to take a deep breath, noting that my own breath had slowed as though to keep pace with him. With the next slow, deep exhalation, I felt nothing but numbness and a wracking body pain al-most as though part of me wanted to jump into the abyss with him so as to not have him go alone. I sat there holding his hand growing colder, wishing I could infuse his body with the warmth of mine. One moment we are of this world, and the next we are not. One moment we know about the fragility and ephemeral essence of life, and the next we do not even know we have lived or that our life meant anything. Only those on this side of that divide know of his having been. And in that moment, I knew that never again would I taste his breath, know his touch, or hear his voice. What was, I knew, would slowly, imperceptibly slip further and further away from my acute sense of his being as our memories fight with grief to hold time still.

Thoughts of having to call my sons and tell them brought me back to this side of life. Then a deafening silence and a muted screaming in my brain. When I finally went home, my youngest son was there and to this day we don't know who held who up. I didn't want to let go, and, finally, in the shower scrubbing as though I could wash off the reality of what had just happened, the tears flowed in the unabashed heaving of my chest and heart. I am quite sure that my son heard my wailing in his room at night. Having been rocklike for me at first, I know that he, too, found his tears that night as well.

The plans we had made, moments of future counted on, suddenly changed. The night he died, I finally slipped into bed with an exhaustion that felt unbearable. I was acutely aware that as I was slipping beneath wakefulness, the emptiness in my stomach and my heart made the bed seem cavernous, welcoming and warning in a Dali-esque sort of way. Although I had been sleeping alone at times when he remained in the living room in his chair too tired and uncomfortable to pretend to sleep in bed, the emptiness of the bed felt now immutable. Rolling from my side to his (does everyone in a couple have a side?), I tried to pretend that both of us were pulling at the comforter to keep the emptiness at bay. I remember awakening with tears and fear propelling me into the shower amid the din of my cries and pain. This was the first day of the rest of my life, and, for now, the beast of grief was my companion for the foreseeable future. When I went downstairs, my younger son was already up, having not slept well himself, and we could do nothing but hold each other and cry. I was acutely aware that, for my youngest son, who had already lost his biological parents as an infant, this loss was something different. As a Mexican American, he and my husband had a special bond around their being people of color, something I could try to understand but not experience. The pain of having lost my own father resurged in my wanting to spare my son the same, but I knew too well that I was powerless to do so.

The ensuing nights brought shadows. Images of old and new parts of our life together dropped in and out of view, disorienting moments in the most vulnerable times of night, intruding on the relief from grief that sleep sometimes gifts. There was no linearity to the intrusive dreams and lucid awakenings. The first few days, surrounded by friends and family by day but alone at night, left me wondering if I could bear it all.

Sitting Shiva

Though my husband was not Jewish, and we were essentially atheistic as a family, we mostly enjoyed the celebratory nature of the major Jewish holidays. We sent out a notice of his passing and held four days of sitting at home, with friends, family, and neighbors stopping by; I was propelled into managing my acute grief by doing what I do best, taking care of everyone else. Friends were attentive, themselves reeling from the loss of a close friend, and the sharing of stories and finding ways to keep him alive made the rawness tolerable, though painful. I felt free to move through tears and laughter, memories of his unique relationships with such a wide diversity of people. But everything I did reminded me of what he could not do, that every thought and feeling shared by those who loved him was lost across the divide between life and death. I reeled in silent rage at the well-meaning but assumptive notion that "he's in a better place." He's nowhere, I screamed inside. Three pounds of jellied neurons stilled, and what of the seventy-one years of life that had been held within? It felt like when I was a child trying to understand what was outside the infinite universe. I searched for wisdom to learn how to say goodbye and bury a lover.

We die with the dying. A piece of us at least. A part of us gets lost: it's the part of the fabric of life knitted and forged in the time together, along with the remnants of each of our pasts. It is that thing we made grew together, not possible to continue alone. With the ending, the cognitive and visceral memories become as objects, "petrified," with all of the meanings of that word. As if to hold the memories, my youngest son built a shrine with pictures, favorite statues, a dim but persistent night light to keep his flame present. With each passing month, new icons landed on the shelves as though to account for the many memories and to keep them from slipping away. I turned to music, tried to play my guitar that was my sanctuary, only to find that some songs we shared elicited too much pain and sadness. Certain words and chord patterns opened floodgates of heaving cries. "If I could save time in a bottle, the first thing that I'd like to do, is to save every day 'til eternity passes away, just to spend them with you." And the existential moment of that part of my own life being over mixed with the reverie of having spent my life intentionally. We pass through time, as Yalom stated: "From one eternity to another."

Thankfully, over weeks, then months, memories of love and pleasure, adventure and calm emerged from the feelings of despair and flooded my waking moments and dreams. Songs we shared from the moment we met, gleaned from boxes of LPs, finding so many duplicated and so many to share that were new to each of us. "Our songs" marked the stages of us growing together, dancing, feeling alive and surprised by the feeling of romance that neither of us had thought was in our nature. Billy Ocean's song "Caribbean Queen" became the unexpected, private reverie:

> Caribbean queen
> Now we're sharing the same dream
> And our hearts they beat as one
> No more love on the run[2]

Sharing friendships made before meeting each other, we grieved together at the National Mall, where we walked with thousands amid the panels of the AIDS Quilt to discover the names of friends with whom we lost touch. Our very lives had been spared by our love together, and though I am forever grateful, we are selfish at the core and always want more. I miss the dance.

It is in my nature to reflect endlessly on my motivations, feelings, and ambivalences: Guilt. Did I push too much? Too little? When he didn't feel like moving after hours of sitting, and I worried that his inactivity was making him even weaker than the cancer, than the medications . . . should I have prodded and pushed more? Rather than simply bear witness to his growing house-boundedness?

Driving. Like the frog who stays in the kettle if you start with cold water and then boils to death, some things creep up unseen, unheard, unfelt. When did he stop going out by himself to the store to pick up this or that? How long had it been since he wanted to drive when we went here or there? When did his dependence on me become so complete?

The boys. I flashed to when I lost my dad. Our boys were different from me and from each other. Adoption made everything different. The older had never really known his father, and at fifteen when he joined our family, he bonded trying to make up for that loss. For the younger, he had already lost his biological parents at birth and had now to face the loss again. Though

I remained, losing his Black father as a Latino young man was different. I did not have the same authority to teach him about the need for caution and the rules of getting through adolescence as a kid of color, the rules and reason for care when wearing a hoodie at night in the streets with his friends. But now he was a grown man, that loss was made complicated as he had also been a major caretaker especially during the past year. To watch my youngest son grow into such a mensch has been an extraordinary gift in the time of such loss. The older boy, however, now in his forties, who had joined our family as a teen, was struggling with his own medical and mental health issues stemming from childhood, unable to participate fully in the grieving process with me, feeling as though he had disappointed us all, and, as he was living elsewhere, was not there to support either me or his brother. Nor could I emotionally gather him in as deeply as I wanted to, trying to protect them both as much as I could from the stabbing pain of my grief. Love is not enough, though at times all we have to give.

Professional Issues

At the time of my loss, I was the Acting Chair of the Department of Psychiatry at one of the Harvard Hospitals, a position I was thrust into rather than chose. Feeling totally untethered to life, I was tempted to resign, unsure about what my absence would mean to the department that was somewhat in disarray. At the same time, I was being urged to apply for the permanent Chair position, something that my husband and I had discussed even before we were in the final stages of his illness. In the midst of trying to regain my footing emotionally and having to let people know that I would be taking some time off to deal with the aftermath of the loss, I had to decide what information to disclose and how to do it. I realized that, had I not been Acting Chair, I would have been very private about my loss and simply said very little. I did feel torn and anxious about leaving an unsettled department uncertain about what had kept me away from work. As the residency program director, I also felt that my thirty-two residents deserved to know why I would suddenly become unavailable to them. Thus, having been used to sending our yearly missives at holiday or other momentous times, I issued a brief but clear statement about my loss and my plan to take a month off. Private grief suddenly made public. I continue to reflect on how our public persona and our private being inform each other, including the ambivalence about however we reconcile the two. I thought about it as a huge sinkhole that begins to grow ever larger, forcing me to step back again as my worlds, private and public, began to feel the same. I came to think that privacy was both protective and harmful and that by being totally open about my experience I would be ironically safer than trying to preserve some sense of control over information or what others thought of me.

Back at work after my husband's death I was struggling to stay focused, to be present; most difficult was trying to think anything was important. I felt so terribly vulnerable in a way I hadn't felt since my own father had died twenty-five years before, when several of my patients knew without my saying anything except "I am away for a week attending to a family emergency and I will contact you when I return." As I did then, I let each of my patients know that I had to postpone our sessions for a personal reason and would call them as soon as I was able to return to work, anticipating at least a month. Even after I returned to work at the hospital, I delayed starting back with my private practice for a few more weeks, deluged with financial and legal processes that seemed surreal at a time of intense mourning. Unending paperwork and meetings, all seeming so futile, part of me screaming inside about the superficial nature of so much of what we encounter in our daily lives. I struggled to find the right posture, the right disclosure, although most of them picked up quickly that I was suffering from something I could not completely hide. What to say, what not to, how to respond to outreaches of caring and love. My patients kept me focused, and they tried to take care of me, often, as I now see it, by minimizing their own feelings and needs. Most difficult was managing my internal experience of one patient who was dealing with the active and prolonged demise of his partner of forty years. I was jealous that he still had someone to worry about, to care for, and though I wanted to scream at him to relish what time he had, I strove to hear his frustrations and fears through the rants about his difficult role. Several times he commented that he felt badly talking about his ill partner knowing about the acute loss of mine. I managed to stumble through with the help of my peers to assure him that I could hear his pain and that I had people taking care of me. Words, appropriate, but empty of the true empathy that was called for. To feel so incompetent and selfish was enough to make me wonder about continuing to do therapy with people, at least in the short term. Slowly, almost four months after my husband's death, I was able to keep the grief at bay for those minutes I had to be in the room with someone in my care.

Then the Ceiling Fell In

Four months after his death, I was still grieving and taking care of the un-ending paperwork and financial sequelae (easier to enter than leave this mortal coil), trying to not make decisions too quickly, trying to make life seem possible for me and the boys. His absence like a huge cavern that had grown in the midst of our house, the floor in the living room opening up as we peered over the edge as if we could see him, or hearing a noise upstairs thinking he was descending the stairs, fooled by the creakiness of a 140-year-old house.

I casually mentioned during a regular exam with my internist who had cared for my husband and me for many years, taking exquisite care of us during his cancer diagnosis and staying with us through the end, that I was having some trouble clearing food at the lower end of my esophagus, what I took to be a metaphor for my internal difficulty in swallowing the reality into which I had been thrust. He, however, took my stomach pain complaint seriously, and, within a couple of days I had a barium swallow and endos-copy, and the pathology report of an adenocarcinoma of the lower esoph-agus. Terror in the midst of grief, my rational defensive mechanisms pushing away the fear to a hyperarousal of organization to prepare for any eventual outcome.

My grieving gave way from worrying about how to survive the loss to wor-rying how to survive at all, and a rapid fear of abandoning my sons surged through me as panic. How was this possible? Even now, there are fleeting moments when I have to remind myself that I actually have had cancer. In the early hours of each morning, alone in bed, awakened by dreams and hallucinations of him being next to me—and then gone and facing my own mortality alone—was frightening. I kept most of that to myself, not wanting to burden my sons. Boundaries, I thought, would allow me to protect them when, in retrospect, I was really protecting myself.

Within weeks I was meeting with my GI cancer treatment team, sorting out the pathology, the options, and mapping my treatment while my own fear strangled my grief. The conversation I had to have with my sons and family made my ability to focus on work nearly impossible. What do I know? What do I say? How do I help my boys hold hope amid uncertainty? The thought that they would lose two fathers within a year was terrifying, and a sense of helplessness overtook my usual coping style to pile through any impediment in my way. A few days of feeling like the ground had opened up beneath me gave way to my "take charge" approach to life, and we sat and planned. I made sure all the paperwork that my younger son would need as my healthcare proxy and power of attorney would leave him empowered to make decisions. As the more responsible of the two boys, and the one living in the house with me, I hated that I had to put him through this preparation in the event I would not survive the treatment. In the details, such as putting his name on the checking account, while acknowledging the possibility that he would have to be in charge, I found some absurdly rationalized sense of control. If I were to die, the paperwork would be in order. I refused to be a burden in death.

Worst was the feeling that I felt the loneliness in my vulnerable state, angry and scared that I would go through this without my husband. (When my youngest son was four, we nightly checked under the bed for those monsters that lurk in the children's literature; at sixty-nine years of age, the monster in the middle of the night was no less real.) As much as my sons were there to support me, they could not be the replacement for someone in the middle of the night when the dark brings our childhood fears into our sleep. This, I realized, was mine to bear, and more than anything it made me reflect on how important, though difficult, it had been for me to be with him in those darkest moments. I sat with the uncertainty for months about whether I would live or die from the cancer.

The defining moment when the fear of annihilation gave way to hope occurred late on a Friday night after having had an abdominal CT scan to stage the cancer. My son sat across from me in the imaging suite, silent, drawing, reminiscent of the many days we sat waiting for my husband to emerge from his scans. The rest of that day was lost, as I thought the weekend would be until I heard about whether I would be cured or die in the not-so-distant future. At 10 P.M. that night the oncologist called me and told me my scan was clean and he said, "You will be cured." He also told me to tell my son, who he called by name, that he wouldn't lose a second father this year. I wept. My son wept, and I wish I could have frozen that hug between us as the panic rushed out of me.

Twenty-nine days of radiation and weekly chemo. Early-morning daily radiation treatments, weekly chemotherapy infusions, and reducing my work schedule to about 75%. Dealing with what to tell my long-term patients and not taking on anyone new without knowing whether I would have time to do the work with them. Once again, the questions about disclosure to patients, staff, and friends. Then waiting until the thorax healed a bit from the radiation until I could undergo surgery. I dove back into work and into spending as much time as I could with my sons. There were moments on the treadmill, elevated to max, as I forced my body to recover, where the mix of feelings brought torrents of tears and pain, fear and anxiety, my heart literally reminding me with every felt beat that I was yet alive, and very much alone.

A bullet dodged. The chemo, radiation, and surgery "cured" the cancer at least for the foreseeable future. I owe my life to my primary care physician and the extraordinary, caring, and dedicated treatment team. By this time, I had gone from 217 pounds down to my college graduation weight of 160, and, for the first time in my life, I had to struggle with maintaining weight. Having to eat almost constantly, scheduling my life around food intake. Gratitude for surviving and discomfort with the burden were ever present. Patients whom I had resumed seeing a month or so after the surgery wanted to ask how I was doing, and did so, often with such respect and caring that I felt compelled to share truthfully about what had happened, sparing details, and letting them know I was planning to be around a while and was surviving the cancer and the treatment. Although known, now felt deeply, the sense of relationships of any kind is the real secret to feeling alive.

When I returned to work, I could feel my residents unsure of how to treat me. Their affection and care were immediately palpable, as was their hesitancy to burden me with what they assumed paled in importance after what I had been through. Their hesitancy troubled me, as, on one hand, it felt extremely loving and protective and, on the other, a reminder of the fragility and vulnerability I actually felt. As is my nature, I told them what I felt and encouraged them to know that I needed them to need me, to see me as present and to bring whatever was on their minds to me, to help me feel alive. I reminded them that what was a real concern of theirs, of whatever magnitude, was important for us to share and that by doing so I would feel useful again. Slowly we have regained the balance of giving and taking.

Compounding the personal issues was the resurgence of grief over my husband's death once I knew I was going to live. I had not anticipated the fury and persistence of its return. Cancer changes the whole story, not only for the individual, with a daily reminder of its impact on the whole of my life and all the people in it. It had put on hold the grieving process for all of us, family and friends who turned their attention to care for me. I do not know where I would be in the grieving process had I not taken ill, nor if it might have been easier or more difficult. I do believe that tasting my own mortality fused my grieving for him with my grieving for me. The finiteness of *my* life, real in the most visceral of ways, was terrifying and eerily comforting in a strange way. I can actually now hold in my mind that I will, if not now, die.

Moving Forward

One year after his death, we had a memorial celebration of his life, bringing together people from so many different parts of his, my, and our life together. Almost all who came knew him in different ways and heard the rounding out of the story of his life with new insights into him and us. The stories were endless, magnificently different, and full of the essence of who he was. I marveled at the different ways he had touched peoples' lives. The following day, a few of us took the fast ferry to Provincetown where he and I had first declared our love and commitment and, in a quiet, private moment, dispersed his ashes into the receding tide until all visible signs of him was taken up by the endless ocean. As with my parents before, water everywhere is a sanctuary for the people I have loved who have loved me.

Two years later, I began accommodating to the change in my life as a single person again. I am a different person because of him. He is gone, I am here, and what we made between us is both still real and ephemeral. The grief remains, daily as the first thought of each morning and the last thought before sleep. Tears remain a moment away, triggered by a memory, a phrase of a poem, a few bars of a song. I eat all day, bits of this and that, trying to maintain my weight as I work out almost daily to regain my strength. I still talk to him aloud; I dream about him. I've had to buy or alter clothes for this new body I have that still feels strange in the mirrored reflection. He liked me "chunky" he used to say: Would he like this new body born out of grief and pain? I hear his reminder about what pieces of clothing go with what. As I dress each morning, I ask myself (and truthfully, him) whether he would have a comment as he often did: "You're wearing *that*?" to which I would often reply, "Apparently not." I have chronicled over and over in my mind the various parts of our relationship I miss and still crave. I miss my lover, my friend, my intellectual sparring partner, my confidant, my professional peer consultant, and my co-parent helping to balance my need for control with my sons' need for autonomy. I ruminate about what happened to all of that stuff inside the three pounds of jellied mass that no longer fires. I read the books he ordered and never got to read, and I talk out loud as though our private book club is still ongoing. I am slowly able to play those songs on my guitar that eluded me, when heaving sighs of grief would wash over me. One of our favorites was by Jim Croce, "Time in a Bottle," with the refrain capturing the truth of how we felt:

> There never seems to be enough time
> To do the things you want to do
> Once you find it.
> I've looked around enough to know
> You're the one I want to go
> Through time with.[3]

Grief is a beast. And the great clarifier. It stops time. It comes in waves. It cleans out the unimportant stuff of day-to-day life while reminding us that the details of living are the essence of life itself. I have come to really understand how working has been so helpful even in the midst of loss and illness. My search for meaning to be part of something larger than me, than him, than us. But there is also an awakening of things yet not done, of places we had hoped to travel that are beginning to beckon me. Suddenly, after fifty years, I returned to the thoughts of what it means for me to be a gay man, now alone, once again somewhat invisible without him by my side. Even my "whiteness," privilege, and experience as a Jew in America feel more complicated without the day-to-day reality and learning of being with a man of color for almost four decades. I treasure the continued embrace by the multicolored family and friends we built. I feel rooted in a vision of the personal world that feels broken right now, but I believe will heal.

I think about how much I will miss him holding me, whispering to me as my time comes to face the abyss. There really is nothing fair or even personal about life. If given the choice, would we ask to be born knowing what might lie ahead? Yet I feel lucky, some would say blessed, that I have loved and been loved, to have had such joy paid for with the price of grief. My grieving is deep, but I have not been depressed. Life still calls for me to let go while holding on. I am beginning to carry the loneliness as proof of love, and while my friends ask about whether I will date(?) again or if I want to find another partner, I know that I am not ready yet to fully, honestly explore that while my grief and recovery from illness is still so much in my mind and heart.

Settling into a new version of one's self is like sculpting with new, never before used tools, and no idea of what the piece will look or feel like. Who am I becoming? What do I do with the ring that now slips off the once fattened finger but refuses to budge: Is it me? Is it him? Will I know when it is time for the ring to come off? I still cannot bear to erase the last voice message I have from him or remove his number from automatic dialing. Can I leave him where he lies in my heart and move on without guilt?

Writing about oneself takes a kind of hubris that has always worried me. Literally billions of people have lived and died, and their stories are not any less new or important than mine. Perhaps every grief lessens with the telling and retelling. I know I could not have managed without my youngest son being by my side throughout. Each of the boys has his own story that is theirs to tell.

Epilogue

Two years and nine months after my husband's death, as I write now. In two weeks, I will meet the two-year mark since my treatment, and I remain cancer free. How is it that time can have such power to keep us simultaneously in the moment of catastrophic loss and propel us forward, moving through grief to a future that becomes now both conceivable and feared for the multiple possibilities, as though one must "get it right?" How does feeling inevitably stuck in a moment of enormous grief, slowly, imperceptibly grow into rejoining the life force that has been there all along, though less attended to in the waves of feeling that loss: fear that we would dishonor the memories and face the loss with insurmountable survivor guilt, cocooned in that grief for eternity. Somehow, perhaps because the life force is stronger than our defenses we emerge, grabbing onto what the living embody and the dead no longer know. The bed is still cavernous and empty, but more mornings than not I awake to feel him both gone and yet very present in the unending memories of our life together. I am not sure that I will ever get to the point where I feel we had enough of life together, but increasingly I feel the gratitude that we had as much time as we did. Thoughts of him bring the impossible combination of joy and sadness in my dreams and waking life. My finger has quietly, remorsefully, released the ring though months later I twirl the phantom band as if to state that, though now alone and visibly so to the world, it will take more time to own my widowhood in all of its dimensions; for the first time, I can imagine waking up with more joy than sadness.

Each life narrative ends in one way, and until that time is worked and reworked, written and rewritten, until our moment in this world ceases with the last breath and beat of our heart. I deeply envy those who have a steadfast belief that they will be reunited with the lost loved ones in their life, but I remain resigned to the stillness that I will share like, but not with, those traveled there before me.

About the Author

Marshall Forstein, MD, is a psychiatrist with more than forty years of experience. He was the co-founder of one of the first HIV Collaborative Care Clinics at the Cambridge Health Alliance (CHA), a public-sector Harvard-affiliated teaching hospital. He has been the Medical Director of Mental Health at the Fenway Health Center, one of the largest health centers dedicated to the LGBTQ communities. For nineteen years, he was the Training Director of the Psychiatry Residency Program at CHA, where he also served as Acting Chair of the Department of Psychiatry and Vice Chair for Education and Training. He has been active on governmental and professional organization committees and task forces in the areas of HIV/AIDS and gender and sexuality and has written and taught nationally. He is currently on the teaching faculty at CHA/Harvard Medical School and maintains a private practice.

Suggested Resources

Songs

Croce, J. (1972). "Time in a bottle." From *You don't mess around with Jim* [audio file]. https://open.spotify.com/track/561F1zqRwGPCTMRsLsXVtL.
Mitchell, J. (1966). "Circle Game." From *Live radio broadcasts*.
Ocean, B., & Diamond, K. (1984). "Caribbean queen (no more love on the run)" [Recorded by B. Ocean]. From *Suddenly* [audio file]. https://open.spotify.com/track/4JEylZNW8SbO4zUyfVrpb7.

Books

Didion, J. (2005). *The year of magical thinking*. New York: Knopf.
Lightman, A. (1992). *Einstein's dreams*. London: Vintage.
Monette, P. (1988). *Love alone: Love alone: Eighteen elegies for Rog*. New York: St. Martin's Press.

References

1 Eliot, T. S. (1942). *Little Gidding*. London: Faber and Faber.
2 Croce, J. (1972). "Time in a bottle." From *You don't mess around with Jim* [audio file]. Retrieved from https://open.spotify.com/track/561F1zqRwGPCTMRsLsXVtL.
3 Ocean, B., & Diamond, K. (1984). "Caribbean queen (no more love on the run)" [Recorded by B. Ocean]. From *Suddenly* [audio file]. Retrieved from https://open.spot ify.com/track/4JEylZNW8SbO4zUyfVrpb7.

12

With This Ring

Cheryl Krauter

No couple buying wedding rings wants to be reminded that someday one of them will have to accept the other one's ring from a nurse or an undertaker.

—Anne Tyler

I lie on the floor holding the still body of my husband in the early hours before the break of an unimaginable dawn that heralds a life without him. The chaos of the earlier storms of paramedics and firemen rushing through the front door and charging into my family room has passed, leaving me behind. I have no memory of them leaving my home after their frantic, helpless efforts to revive John. The whole scene is taking place like a nightmare, only this is real and I will not awaken, sweating and sighing with the relief that it is only a dream. In this shattering reality, I am gasping for air, my body is shaking, my teeth are rattling. I have fallen into an interior world that is like a dark tunnel without light; I hear the distant sound of myself wailing.

An eerie stillness surrounds me as my wailing has now become streams of tears falling onto his naked chest. There is no longer a beating heart to feel, only a vague sense of the presence of a shattered heart that has burst apart, leaving him dead in less than five minutes. All that wildness, the turmoil of large men stomping through the house, the sounds of "clear, clear" as hands on a defibrillator try to shock John back into life are now only echoes in my mind. My fingers discover a remnant of a failed rescue attempt in a small adhesive patch still stuck to his chest. I remove it gently, delicately, concerned not to hurt him. It's still unreal that he is dead, that he feels nothing, and I suddenly feel like a crazy woman. What world am I in? Aloud, I keep repeating to no one, "What am I going to do, what am I going to do?" I remain with him, talking to him, asking questions that he cannot respond to, stroking his head.

In the distance I hear another knock at the front door that announces the arrival of two mortuary men. I have no memory of calling them. Did I call them, or did someone else? I don't know. I don't want to let them in. These men do not arrive in a hurry, there is no flurry of activity, only their grim but kind faces looking at me as I open the door and allow them in. Just like in the movies, they wear black suits, white shirts, and skinny black ties. They do not bring instruments of resuscitation, they offer no hope of a miracle, they are the agents of the Grim Reaper who has already arrived and then flown away into an unbearable darkness. They bring with them the objects of departure, a gurney and a large black body bag for my husband's final departure. I want to slam the door in their pale, concerned faces.

"Hello," one of them says to me.

"Hello," I mumble back.

As I open the door, the other man asks, "where is the body?'

Oh my God . . .

I walk them back to the room to find John. It is both the longest and shortest distance I have ever traveled. As one of them unfurls the black bag, I begin to shake again. I want them to take him back to the bedroom and put him back in bed, not wrap him in a thick, black bag whose zipper suddenly resembles a horrifyingly enormous, shiny pair of jaws. All three of us are looking down at John's body on the floor. My knees buckle and I sink down to sit beside him.

"Would you like his wedding ring?" one man asks.

"Oh, yes, yes, I would," I manage to choke in a strangled voice I barely recognize as my own.

As the man kneels beside me to remove John's ring, I am transported back to the day when our wedding rings were created.

I am seeing John, young and dark-haired, standing by the eccentric artist who was his jewelry teacher, his white wispy hair blowing in the breeze, skinny arms protruding from a ripped white tee shirt. He'd commonly introduce himself as Bob . . . with one "o." Younger myself, long black curls falling past my shoulders, I stand watching them prepare the casting procedure for the wedding rings that John, himself a jewelry designer, has created for us. The day is sweltering, and it doesn't help that we are standing by the heat of a torch whose flame will melt pieces of gold into liquid that will be poured into a mold to be fired in the nearby flaming hot kiln.

The ounces of gold are placed into a crucible, a ceramic container for melting metal at an extremely high temperature. A crucible is also a situation of severe trial, one in which different elements interact, leading to the creation of something new. Both alchemical: one substance, one form becomes another, transforms what once was into something new. I watch the pieces of gold meld into a stunning river of flowing golden liquid. I quietly observe the breathtaking process, witnessing the molten, brilliant stream being poured into a mold that will hold it, form it, into two wedding rings that are being created in the shape of the symbol for infinity. It is a day when infinity seems possible.

I awake from this dream-like memory as the mortuary man holds out the gold infinity band and places it in my hands. I look at my hands and see my ring still in its place on my finger, John's lays in the palm of my hand. This morning, infinity is ephemeral.

"We don't recommend that you watch this," the man tells me when it is time to move John into his death shroud. I stumble into the living room. I realize that I don't know these men's names; they are merely nameless boatmen crossing over the River Styx, carrying my husband off only to place him into a small, freezing container less than five miles from our home. Far too quickly I hear the wheels of the gurney approaching and watch in a frozen state of disbelief as it is rolled out the door taking John away forever.

I wander from room to room, breathless with sobs. I begin to sink into a watery world, a timeless place that I have never known. In one shattering moment the ground beneath me has shaken and opened up into a crevasse, and I am frightened that I will sink into an unrecognizable darkness from which I will not find my way back. A sudden death, the jagged edges of a disappearance that has no warning, surrounds me like a fog rolling in, leaving nothing visible except a dense, gray mist that envelopes me. I cannot see anything in front of me.

"What am I going to do?"

"What am I going to do?'

These first moments of the sudden loss of John left me stunned. Eventually, I began to surface from beneath the waves of grief, coming up for air, trying to find my way. But, unlike the shock that swiftly knocked me over, it took a while to find the ground beneath my feet once again. I wandered through the world in a dreamlike state. Days faded into weeks and months as the world continued on, uncaring of the loss I was struggling with. Living in this timeless state, I have no memory of the point in time after John died when I decided to remove my own wedding ring. I don't remember how I got to the choice, only that at some point I said to myself, "I can't be married to a dead man." And now, how to get this off my finger!

One darkening fall evening, I light a candle and sit quietly, alone with a deep sorrow, an ache in my chest, as I contemplate taking off this golden ring of infinity. I feel myself releasing another layer of the loss of John, our marriage, the years spent together. As I weep, I begin covering my finger with mountains of hand cream until my whole hand is so slippery that it's hard to get much traction on the ring. Twisting and turning it, I almost had it over my knuckles until it got stuck. By now the finger was not only greasy but swollen up like a sausage, making any progress impossible. My sad ritual came to an unsuccessful conclusion and a sore finger.

I went to the internet to research how to get a ring off. My methods included looping a string between my finger and the ring, applying copious amounts of olive oil, and then tugging the thread. I was left with another enlarged, oil-slicked, red and puffy finger. I tried ice. I tried dental floss. I used plastic wrap. The continued agony of dealing with the ring paralleled the anguish within me. I wanted this whole thing to be over, I didn't want to look down at a symbol of the loss I was struggling with, which now seemed mirrored in futile attempts at the removal of the painful reminder that I was now a widow.

When death strikes suddenly, the aftershocks can be surprising both in their intensity and unpredictability. After my useless, miserable attempts at getting my ring off, I start to recognize the fact that I am actually going to need to have it cut off of my finger. I feel so sad, so vulnerable as I contemplate having my wedding ring sliced apart, the circle of a promise broken. I find a local jewelry store, ask if they can cut off a ring, and, when told yes, make a time to go.

Arriving at the upscale store, I remember other venues where John's jewelry was once displayed. Did he ever show here? All the galleries, the shows, and images of his gorgeous creations flood my mind as I walk into this place. I feel shaky, my voice sounds thin and unsteady as I interrupt the inane chatter of the two women behind the display case with my request. This is a far cry from my original attempt at a sacred ring-removing ritual. The women glance knowingly at me, then snigger a bit as they nod at one another and then back at me. Do they not notice that I am unsmiling, pale, wobbly?

"Oh," one of the women says, "We've done this quite a few times."

"Yes," the other chimes in, "it's wonderful to be able to help someone move on."

They assume that I am surely in the process of a nasty divorce and will be relieved to be rid of the reminder of a dastardly spouse whom I am glad to have out of my life. My response, telling them that I am a widow, created a stillness like frost on a winter window pane. One of the women brings out a tool that will cut metal but not flesh, and we are all silent. In the end, they do not charge me for the service. I leave the shop with my severed wedding ring and drive home alone.

The final resting place of the two rings is in a small, open black velvet ring box next to John's picture. The ring that is cut nestles up against the ring that is still whole. One circle broken, the other forever a sphere of infinity, they touch one another in a light embrace. As I continue in my solitary life, I find myself rubbing the indentation on my finger that is still slender from my wedding ring. I am grateful to touch this circle of skin around my finger as

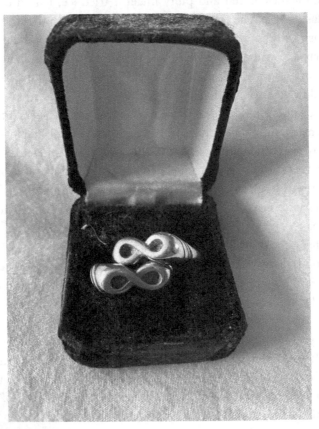

Two Rings

it reminds me that, even in profound absence, there is healing. Within me grows a deepening understanding that a broken ring, like a broken heart, is a beautiful memory of a life and an infinite love.

About the Author

Cheryl Krauter, MFT, is an Existential Humanistic psychotherapist with more than forty years of experience in the field of depth psychology and human consciousness. Her extensive background in theater arts, working with performing artists, visual artists, and creative people, has inspired her to integrate these skills into her therapeutic interventions. She works with people who have been diagnosed with cancer and other life-threatening illnesses, their partners, family members, and caregivers. She has published three books: *Surviving the Storm: A Workbook for Telling Your Cancer Story* (Oxford University Press 2017); *Psychosocial Care of Cancer Survivors: A Clinician's Guide and Workbook for Providing Wholehearted Care* (Oxford University Press 2018); and *Odyssey of Ashes: A Memoir of Love, Loss, and Letting Go* (She Writes Press 2021).

Ms. Krauter maintains private practices in both Albany and San Francisco, California. She is a former board member of the Women's Cancer Resource Center in Oakland, California. She is also a practicing therapist and workshop presenter with the Free Therapy Program. Ms. Krauter has developed workshops and courses and has presented her important work nationally at the American Psychosocial Oncology Society, the Cancer Support Community, and the Northern California Group Psychotherapy Society, among others. She is the co-founder of Savvy Survivor, an online resource for cancer survivors, at www.savvysurvivor.net.

Suggested Resources

Movies

Bender, L. (Producer), & Van Sant, G. (Director). (1997). *Good Will Hunting* [motion picture]. United States: Miramax.
Brooks, J. L. (Producer, Director). (1983). *Terms of Endearment* [motion picture]. United States: Paramount Pictures.

Rivera, J. (Producer), & Doctor, P. (Director). (2009). *Up* [motion picture]. United States: Pixar Animation Studios.

Books

Green, J. (2012). *The Fault in Our Stars*. New York: Penguin Group.
Kalanithi, P. (2016). *When Breath Becomes Air*. New York: Random House.

Songs

MacColl, E. (1969). "The First Time Ever I Saw Your Face" [recorded by R. Flack]. From *First Take* [audio file]. Retrieved from https://open.spotify.com/track/0SxFyA4FqmE QqZVuAlg8lf

Parton, D. (1983). "I Will Always Love You" [recorded by K. Roberts]. From *Eyes That See in the Dark* [audio file]. Retrieved from https://open.spotify.com/track/7mZAKum GUOkskgrIzbdF46

13

Good Times, Brother

John Halporn

The story of my brother's cancer divides my life into a "time before" and a "time after," as a person and as a physician.

My younger brother Doug called me with his biopsy results from the hospital in Burlington, Vermont, several days after undergoing surgery. I imagined him there, wearing his plaid flannel pajamas: thin, wiry, muscular, sitting in a recliner with his feet up on the hospital bed fiddling with the phone cord. He was thirty-four, a fourth-year medical student, a husband, and the father of a one-year-old-daughter. *"They are saying it is a primary gastric cancer stage II. I'll probably need chemotherapy and radiation. But I feel much better, and this morning I ran up twenty flights of stairs for the fun of it."*

In October of that year, he started having unusual-smelling burps—his medical team even noticed the odd sulfur smell one day during patient rounds. A month later, while preparing for Thanksgiving, he became unable to eat or drink anything without vomiting. We had talked about the burps, but, despite our regular calls, he said nothing about feeling full and nauseated long after eating; much later, he told me he had known and felt that something was wrong for several months. He was admitted, scoped, and prepared for surgery to remove what was presumed to be an obstructing stomach ulcer—an unusual diagnosis, but still the most likely explanation in an otherwise healthy young person.

The initial report, after his otherwise successful surgery, was "suspicious for malignancy," and we awaited the final results with hope and dread. He called from his hospital room that day, hours before he was to return home, and told me about the results and the stair climbing. I said, "I love you, and I'll be with you no matter what happens." I felt disbelief, thinking of this news as the worst possible explanation for his situation and wishing to protect him from what I knew to be its ominous meaning. Based on his stage of disease, the five-year survival rate was less than 30%.

I think my pledge on the phone scared him more than reassured him, with its implication of harder times to come and more disappointment to unpack from the results. The report of running the stairs seemed more important to him than the pathology; I wondered if he was purposefully distracting himself or just didn't want to face the truth. Also, he didn't really know much about this disease; unfortunately, I knew more than I would have liked at that moment: it is rarely curable, it brings terrible intestinal symptoms, and the treatments are long and difficult. I knew he could not continue the life he loved. Everything must—and would—change.

I remember putting the phone down and sitting at the top of the stairs at our house in Maine. I shrieked, "Dougie's going to die" and sobbed. There was a stabbing feeling in my chest from the reflexive medical judgment that he would die from this. I had completed my internal medicine training two years earlier, and I was a busy primary care doctor. My fiancée and housemate comforted me, reminding me that we didn't know the whole story yet and that Doug was remarkably hardy. She, too, seemed reassured by his running the stairs. I was certain that a stomach cancer with two involved lymph nodes was not curable and could only be temporarily suppressed with even the best available treatments. It was just a matter of time, I thought: a year, maybe two.

Doug and I were connected so deeply that, in a way, I felt what he felt; just a look between us would do to confirm, with no words necessary. Once, when I visited him in Africa during his Peace Corps assignment in Niger, a mostly desert country in West Africa, we were riding his government-issued motor bike from his village into the capital city of Niamey. My chest was pressed to his back, my arms encircled him, and our helmets kept bumping as we bounced along the parched sandy road. We were passed by a huge motorcycle driven by a figure clad head-to-toe in black leather and helmet. His motorcycle was barely idling as he went by. Doug revved his little engine and we squeaked by this desert biker—we each gave him an overconfident wave before he accelerated and disappeared ahead of us. This is how we felt together—strong, silly, adventurous, and full of joy. This embrace was and is the best moment of our lives together. Now, I wondered how many moments we had left.

Doug, two years younger, and I had many such adventures together: traveling, camping, hiking, skiing, cycling, and sailing. We always fell into an easy rhythm the minute we saw each other, no matter how much time had passed. Once, on a canoe trip in the Adirondacks, before he left for Africa, we had to paddle upstream for five days before we reached this remote beautiful lake dotted with gigantic ancient pine trees rising hundreds of feet from the water. We arrived at sunset, and I can see Doug at the bow of the canoe smiling in the alpenglow, exhausted and exhilarated after the long haul to get there. We turned around the next day and covered the same distance back in just one day. Every day we sang songs, reveled in the beautiful fall foliage and light, and even ate wild cucumbers we found growing at our campsites. We talked the whole time—six straight days—about growing up, our parents, love, meaning, God, life.

We had been apart for several years before his illness; I was in Cleveland, Ohio, in medical school, and he was away for two years in the Peace Corps. We each wrote about a hundred letters over this time, and, after I visited, we adopted greetings and farewells in Fulfuldi, the language of his village— *"Say jam neewala, Love Doug"* ended his letters. After we both returned East, we resumed our monthly visits and frequent phone calls. He told me about returning to our "fast-paced materialistic world" and musing about his girlfriend and a future career. I described what I was seeing and feeling immersed in medicine training. He was my best friend.

There were ways I was helpful immediately after his surgery. I explained the situation gently to our elderly parents and relatives. *"Doug is free of cancer for now, but he needs treatment to prevent recurrence and even the best treatment has uncertain success."* I arranged a consultation at a cancer center in Boston where his proposed treatment was strongly endorsed. I helped Doug talk through his chemotherapy and radiation options and how he might juggle the completion of his medical school requirements. He would find a way a way to finish his fourth year on time by choosing his electives and vacation time during the hardest parts of treatment.

Once that winter we went to Mount Mansfield, our favorite ski area. He was a gazelle on his telemark skis; everyone on the slope turned to watch his agile, graceful movement. We stopped for our usual McDonald's French fries on the way home. As he took the bag from the drive-through window, he gave me his goofy smile—early crow's feet and wide toothy grin on his thin stubbly face—and chuckled, "Good times, brother." This was "I love you," "I love us," and "I love life" combined.

I became a tireless advocate, pushing Doug and his providers to address every detail and to be direct in their communication about benefits and burdens. It was uncomfortable being the assertive "doctor-brother," and I watched his oncologist and nurse wince when I spoke up. There is a way that doctors like to tie up the plan as though it is agreeable to all; I would describe to Doug that he had more choices than he was hearing or being offered. *"You could also start your chemotherapy this week on Friday instead of next Tuesday; Fridays will work much better with your school schedule."* It was so clear to me how he should be treated, with all options presented and enough time to consider his best choices. I thought there was only one way, and I tried to push until it happened, thinking I was securing the right care for him. Doug told me to "back off" at several points; many times, my partner encouraged me to "let go" and allow things to proceed on their own in Vermont and check in several days later. I knew he needed me to let go at times, I was intrusive and inflexible, yet letting go left me feeling numb and empty.

I kept a greater distance after he recovered from surgery as I felt it was important for Doug and his family to be independent and self-sufficient. I suffered with frustration and helplessness, however, hearing about the false starts and circular communication in his treatment. One example: deciding how soon after the surgery Doug could begin radiation and chemotherapy required a conversation between his oncologist and surgeon, and both Doug and I tried by phone for a week to facilitate this. It wasn't until these two providers had a chance meeting in the hospital parking garage several days later that they could come to agreement. In the end we didn't lose any time, but the process was haphazard and infuriating to me. I considered it evidence of less than adequate attention and caring from his providers. It would take me several years to appreciate that this is the human experience of complex illness—repetition of information, clumsiness in communication, false starts, and the continual refinement of common understanding. It would take much time and experience yet for me to see that perfectly delivered logistics and problem-solving was not the same as the understanding and empathy that I wanted for him at that time.

Doug finished his treatment in the spring of his last year of medical school, completed his final requirements, was matched in a residency training program, and graduated on time. What a superstar. He even spoke at his graduation about his experience with cancer in great detail, down to the repeated denials of coverage from his school-sponsored health insurance. This gap in coverage was rectified, but Doug expressed how much this added to the stress of being gravely ill. I was so proud of him, and I admired his unvarnished reflection on illness: he was going to be a wonderful doctor. During the speech, our Dad realized for the first time that Doug may not have survived his surgery and treatment and that his future was still uncertain. It was one of the two times I saw our father speechless and in tears; the other time would be at Doug's funeral three grueling years later. Doug was thinner now, wearing a sharp blue suit, and holding his one-year-old with an arm around his wife. My mother couldn't stop smiling and taking pictures. It was the last time our whole family would be together without a sense of dread for Doug's future.

Doug and his wife made the difficult decision to defer his residency training; they wisely opted to stay in Vermont, focusing on Doug's health and their thriving daughter instead of relocating and starting the grueling work schedule that awaited him as an intern. He spent that year being a father, tutoring anatomy, and working for his local ambulance service. His tasks were to maintain his medical knowledge and skills and earn some income to help support his family. It was his last good year: he felt well, held his weight, and had his best ski season ever. *Doug, how many days did you ski this week dude? Only four, bro.*

I made many changes during this year as well. My fiancée and I were married in the summer, and Doug looked strong and healthy standing up as my best man. Same blue suit, but a little more filled out and tanned from a summer outside—he smiled the whole weekend and his pride in me was palpable. I finished my primary care job, and we arranged to move back to Boston where I would work as a hospitalist. I visited Vermont less than monthly, and I was relieved to see Doug and family return to a regular rhythm and self-sufficiency. He was the primary homemaker, working in his garden, driving his daughter to school, and preparing meals. His life was rich and full of meaning.

As I prepared to leave my medical practice in Maine before our move, I was pleased and surprised by the gratitude from my well-known patients. Two older men who had given me pointers as a beginning woodworker made me beautiful handmade gifts for my office which I still treasure. I realized that I had been special to them; now I see that it was not for the efficient care but for the connection and friendship we had developed.

I found an intensive palliative care education and practice course at Harvard Medical School that would begin in the month before I began as a hospitalist—I was eager to learn more after using some of the skills in my practice and seeing the tremendous need with my brother. Palliative care as a practice and specialty had not arrived at many medical institutions in 2001, and certainly not in Vermont, where my brother was treated. In Doug's case, absent were the opportunities for conversations with his surgeon and oncologist (or palliative care physician) about prognosis, coping with illness and uncertainty, and clarifying Doug's hopes and fears about his disease. He would have made the same choices for aggressive treatment, but with a more concrete understanding of situation and future. This understanding and dialogue would have brought him an increased feeling of control and support: I was sad to learn what he might have had.

Doug finished the year after his graduation feeling well and with reassuring scans. Again, I worried more than he did, knowing the window for cancer recurrence remained open. The worry was a nagging feeling or a snide voice saying, "don't get too comfortable, this isn't over." Following the advice of my medical colleagues, I convinced Doug and his providers to perform a surveillance endoscopy in May before his internship started in late June. I called him that morning and told him I loved him, again pledging that I would help him with whatever happened. He mentioned their plans for a celebratory hike that afternoon once the sedation wore off. I scared him a second time I realized; unfortunately, the pledge and fear were prescient.

The endoscopy showed local progression of tumor in his remaining stomach. He moved quickly to a full gastrectomy, removing the last of his stomach and connecting his esophagus to the small intestine. His official prognosis and disease stage did not change, and he did not require more treatment, yet his life changed dramatically with this second surgery. Eating, digestion, and nutrition all became difficult; too much, too fast, or the wrong balance of foods caused nausea, colic, sweats, and lightheadedness. He loved to eat, and he and his family grieved this loss of enjoyment and togetherness. After eating he would recline in his chair, breathe heavily, sweat, and moan quietly. It was a small house and sound carried—all three of them became increasingly anxious.

There was helpful distraction from the difficult time with Doug and his family as my wife and I prepared for new jobs and a new home. We longed to return to the city and a faster pace of life. I had to miss the final work of moving to Boston while helping Doug through surgery; my wife and mother-in-law completed this mountain of effort, for which I am forever grateful.

Privately, I grieved Doug's losses, knowing his life was now irreparably different and his beautiful, muscular body had been radically altered by disease, surgery, chemotherapy, and radiation. His hard-won pounds of muscle that he regained after the first round disappeared in weeks—his clothes were so loose that he wore suspenders and bulky sweaters to keep warm. His face, too, lost the weathered tan; his cheeks began to thin—ever so slightly, each visit for the next two years. I dreaded seeing the change when I arrived, and I tried to "save" and savor his appearance as I left.

The palliative care course was challenging, coming so close on the heels of Doug's setback, but I was also fascinated by the depth and meaning of the work. Primary was using language, nonverbal behaviors, time, and silence to form a connection with the patient; I knew this feeling from my practice to date, but here was an opportunity to use the connection therapeutically and gain some confidence from the examples and experience of others. The overriding belief in the patient as the empowered center of medical care and the work of clarifying and honoring what he or she understood and wanted were values and practices I shared. These are important to all types of medical practice, but they are the central aim and process of palliative care. This felt right to me as a doctor and as the brother of a patient.

The knowledge and style I learned answered my need for honesty and deep caring, and I had inklings of the doctor I wanted to be—compassionate, knowledgeable, comprehensive—a witness to my patients' struggles and a trusted partner. The experience built on my four years in practice and gave me practical knowledge that assisted in my brother's illness. While there, I made important connections that allowed me to become an informal palliative care fellow at Dana Farber Cancer Institute in addition to my hospitalist practice.

I held a great deal of loneliness at the same time; my powerful grief left me unable to share my experience and vulnerability and its effect on my work— even among this group of patient and empathetic people. I felt pressure and fluttering in my chest and unsteady on my feet when I spoke tangentially about it—I would collapse if I said more. I listened as others were able to talk about their grief from personal and professional loss and how they had incorporated this into their practice. I envied the ability to be so open; it felt too raw for me, and, despite pushing myself to speak, I always turned back. I would not be ready to share my experience with peers for several years, but I could feel it, waiting and wanting to come out. It was clear that palliative care doctors were a reflective lot, and many had come to this field after overcoming significant personal loss and experiencing devasting patient tragedies. Some part of me knew it was the right place for me.

Within weeks of his surgery, Doug started his family medicine internship. He was ecstatic about being a physician; he ordered a Vermont vanity plate for his car—DOC2BE. *Well, if it isn't Doc Tubey!* He worked with his usual indomitable spirit and performed very well, but within two months it became apparent that he could not sustain the pace. He had three bouts of pneumonia, and he slowly lost weight. We hoped it was simply fatigue and not enough time to assemble and eat his restricted diet. He was failing and ignoring it stubbornly; it was terrible to see his shrinking muscles and accumulating exhaustion.

Over those months as he tried to keep up with his healthy colleagues, I reduced my work hours to spend more time as a caregiver in their house—helping with errands and appointments, cooking, cleaning, and shopping, all while Doug worked. One of the joys for me was playing with my niece, who was three and thriving with the increased adult attention and a new school. She was proud of her daddy as a doctor and did not seem to know about his surgery and changed eating.

By November, Doug's condition had worsened; he now had constant nausea, abdominal pain, and bloating. He developed a bowel obstruction in early December. This time the surgery was not so simple; he had diffuse abdominal cancer and a "frozen" abdomen, meaning his intestines were so adhesed that he lost all motility. He awoke with an ileostomy and began an unreal existence: daily IV nutrition (TPN) instead of eating and weekly suppressive chemotherapy to retard further spread of cancer. He was devasted by the loss of his work and identity as a physician and unsure of how much time he had left. His surgeon intimated that a comfortable Christmas might be the most he could hope for.

I hoped I was performing well as a hospitalist and palliative care fellow at the time; I lost myself in the immediacy of complex patient care and engaging colleagues. The now raging doctor-brother came out both at work and with Doug's caregivers, however. Injustice and incomplete patient care were sensations, a visceral clenching and restlessness, prompting me to proclaim and sometimes rant about our obligation to patients and the need for better caring. *Perhaps if you paid more attention to the patient after you finished your procedure, we would not have to delay his discharge while you decide where he should be followed!* My colleagues generally agreed with my logic, but they were also fearful of my reactions. I felt isolated; no one else acted this way, and the frequency and degree of conflict was unpleasant for all of us. I did not feel much internal restraint once triggered, and I worried how far I might go. Was I alone in my judgments and betrayed by my instincts?

With his usual fortitude, Doug did better than anyone expected after this surgery. He settled into a routine of rest, chemotherapy, and artificial nutrition, and he spent his available energy with his wife and daughter. We had one last adventure that spring: skiing in Alta, Utah, his all-time favorite mountain. This is in a narrow steep valley filled with snow and summits in all directions. There is a quiet hush from the constant wind and an absence of human sound. The sun was warm, the sky a deep blue, the nights were very dark, and the snow was brilliant white and everywhere. The adventure was tempered by the ravages of illness. His wife and daughter needed a break from his care, and they decided to stay home at the very last minute. Doug contended with nightly TPN and daily IV antibiotics while we were there; he tried unsuccessfully to go in the outdoor pool—stopped by the flimsy cover on his ostomy bag and the dressing over his chest IV port. There were moments as a gazelle on skis with glimpses of his former power and grace, but he was tired and weak most of the time and it showed. His stylish ski outfit looked too big on him, his usual cocky roll walking in ski boots was gone, and his face was pale and tired. He was happy to be there, but sad about his loss of prowess; he was no longer master of the terrain. He cracked his biggest smile of the trip one evening when we photographed him on the snowy hotel room balcony in a recliner, TPN bag and tubing hanging from his crossed skis, a cold beer in one hand and a thumbs-up in the other. He never explained how or why he mustered such strength at moments like this; like his previous mastery on the ski slope, it was plain to see. At work, I continued my outspoken patient advocacy, but my eloquence remained hollow and disruptive. I did not make a significant change in the caring and commitment of our institution; I simply altered the paths of my few patients. This made a difference, often very significant, for these individuals, but using methods of nearly intolerable conflict and stress. My training with two senior palliative care clinicians began to help me let go of the ownership I felt over outcomes; I needed to lose the feeling of personal failure and unworthiness. I started to believe that presence and intention were far more important than a perfect medical transaction. It was also intensely rewarding—I felt closer to my patients as people and more valuable in what I brought to their care and to their lives. This was a glimpse of who I could be.

Doug failed slowly over the next year with progressive fatigue and weight loss, suffering gradual liver failure and deep jaundice, complications from long-term TPN. He talked less over his last year, from exhaustion and his preoccupation with the next feeding or medication. He always chose the available treatments to stay alive for his wife and daughter, but his existence was mostly sleeping, being incompletely awake, and always tired. We watched a lot of TV; episodes of Madeline the French orphan cartoon were something of obsession for both Doug and his four-year-old daughter. I became even closer with my niece—I knew her preschool teachers and friends, I played "let's get married" hundreds of times (I was the groom,) and I comforted her and put her to bed more often than Doug did.

I could see Doug in my sick patients then, particularly young people with cachexia. I understood the incredible effort needed sometimes just to roll over or speak. I saw their irritability with any effort and the agonizingly slow passage of time. I learned to sit at eye level and be silent, to be a witness, and to use the silence and power of witness as an essential component of my care. Doctoring felt like work, like lifting a heavy weight, letting some of the patient's despair and exhaustion wash over me. I was not sure at first that bearing witness was enough. Was I being proactive? I was not actively doing anything. My mentors assured me this very silence was essential to caring. *You have a warm presence with your patients, they trust you.* Patients were comforted when I returned to see them a second or third time.

In June 2003, Doug was having trouble climbing the stairs to his bedroom and was too exhausted to connect his TPN, missing some nights, which led to increased listlessness the following day. His wife and daughter were suffering too—skipping meals, both losing weight, and spending more time away from the house because of the grim silence with Doug at home. They had talked about a nearby hospice house, but they were not ready to move him. I finally told Doug he had to go: his family was suffering, and his care needs were too great. Neither of us wanted this, but we both understood that he had to for his family—for their ability to stay living in the house and to recover from his approaching death. His wife protested mightily; luckily, her friends converged and convinced her as well.

Although dreading his death, I was ready for Doug's life to be over. I was also sad and exhausted, and I resented missing much of the nesting at home as we prepared for the birth of our first child.

Doug was placed in a rabbit-themed pediatric room at the hospice house, ten minutes from their home. My four-year-old niece was happy about his "bunny room." He was prepared: he planned his funeral service, recorded a short speech for all of us, and decided who he wanted at his bedside when his final moment arrived. He was comfortable and mostly sleeping, one of the last things he noticed was the rich smell from a volunteer roto-tilling the garden outside. He died after a week in the hospice house, in the evening, with several of us there while his chosen Bing Crosby Christmas album played. It was June, and the windows were open—the garden's earthy aroma and the sound of crickets wafting in—he took a last quiet breath and left us.

The funeral was two weeks later in his local church. The minister knew him well and gave a very personal eulogy, his many friends and neighbors filled every seat. Our dad spoke and gave a sad description of losing a son,

I sang a folk song about the historic town where we grew up. There was relief that the physical suffering was over, and we could close this chapter of our lives; the funeral was the last little step. It all seemed quite far away—people's condolences and hugs perfunctory and not coming close to recognizing the last three and a half years.

Life moved quickly for me then. Our daughter was born a month later, I changed to a less intense job, still as a hospitalist but now much closer to home. I carried Doug's ID badge at work under my own, clipped to my left breast pocket, as reminder and remembrance. The raging at "incomplete" care worsened at first, from both my wounds and the increased distance from the academic center and the influence of palliative care. My awareness of imperfection meant my complicity—I worked and railed tirelessly. Again, a few were helped, some individual cases maybe, but the institution and colleagues did not change, and my efforts probably worsened the physician atmosphere at my small community hospital.

Time, experience, and therapy ultimately drove me to change in order to become the physician I wanted to be. Over the next ten years I gradually evolved, along with job changes and conversion to solely palliative care practice. I had an excellent counselor who helped me slowly unpack and reflect on the rush of experiences of the three years of Doug's illness and death. *Much of the universe is beyond our control, even beyond our awareness,* he might say. Or *a person is like a house with all the doors and windows wide open. Events, thoughts, and feelings just blow in and out; we should simply observe them. It is the awareness and intention that matter.* These were the right messages for me, although it has taken time to absorb them, years really. I miss my brother every day, even now, the friend I cannot call, someone who thinks I am funny, and I carry my family memories just by myself. Some moments have been deeply sad: the deaths of our parents, our children growing up, the dreams we had about traveling and retiring next door to each other.

This writing has helped me understand and accept myself a little better—I have pain in the recalling and describing, but when I finish a draft there is relief and a bit more distance from the hurt. I recognize the two angles I have focused on: what happened and how I reacted and adapted. The first is an effort to accurately record and honor our life-changing experience. The second is the work of accepting how I was and how I am. I feel some shame in my behavior—I was very difficult many times—forgiving myself for this imperfect humanness is where I have learned the most. I can quickly detect similar pain in others despite their thick armor and difficult behavior; over time, as

I work with them, I learn about the feelings underneath and know how to provide comfort. I realize that I am not done writing, and this is not the entire story, as threads of it have yet to occur and some are still too sensitive to be exposed.

There is no sweetness in the lessons I take from Doug's illness, but I have learned a great deal. I can now be the patient older physician who listens to patients and colleagues; I reflect on the immediate morass we are in and create a way forward. Much of what I do is make the delivery of bad news more direct and understandable, often deepening the immediate sadness and despair. But I know that the honesty and compassion are right and in the correct balance. I feel it through the tears of families, patients, and colleagues. The righteousness still comes out sometimes, too much for my liking, but I think it is more constructive. I can recognize it sooner, often in the moment; I apologize and join with the "accused" most of the time. Humor and humility help soften the sharp edges.

The obligation to honor Doug's tragedy and suffering is strong and always near the surface. It is not joyful, but a need and a presence that I feel daily. I do it for him and for myself. I think he would be proud of me.

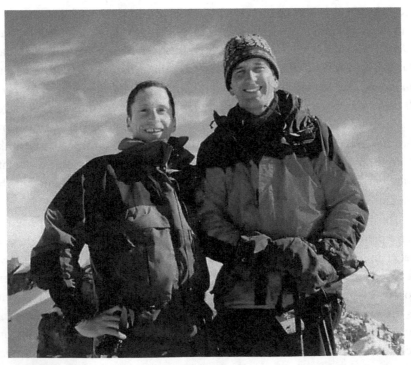

Alta Utah 2000, author at right

About the Author

John Halporn, MD, is a palliative care doctor and internist. He began his practice as a primary care doctor in Maine and then spent 10 years as a hospitalist and hospitalist program director before changing to full time palliative care practice and teaching. He currently works at Brigham and Women's Faulkner Hospital, Dana-Farber Cancer Institute, and Care Dimensions Hospice. He is Director of the Harvard Practical Aspects of Palliative Care CME Course.

14

For Better or for Worse

A Couple Reconfigures Life After Loss

Joan Heller Miller and Ken Miller

Ken

The story started for me in 1976, at Tufts University. I was crazy about Joan the first time I met her. I admired her beautiful face and dark/light curly hair as she played her guitar and sang Joni Mitchell's "Circle Game." I loved the sweet smell of her breath, and anticipated seeing her as I walked to her dorm room and smelled her perfume.

After that first meeting, we were married four years later. It is difficult to compress our three-dimensional life onto the two-dimensional page. I was a resident physician in internal medicine and Joan, a mental health practitioner, was helping obese children develop a healthier lifestyle. Life was busy and fulfilling.

Our oldest daughter Cara was born in 1984, an added joy to our lives. At six months, I knew that something wasn't right, and an audiologist confirmed profound hearing loss. As a new parent, I sobbed: Would Cara learn to talk, would she have friends, would she become a successful and happy adult? The pediatrician was correct in saying that our "lives would never be the same."

Julie, our second child, born in 1988, unexpectedly at age eight started to develop early puberty. A brain MRI did not reveal a brain tumor, but rather a rare fluid collection in the spinal cord: a condition called syringomyelia. We got multiple expert second (or third) opinions, with each one slightly different and contradictory. Ultimately, we took our little Julie to Chicago for planned surgery and she had a preop MRI. The surgeon popped his head into the waiting room and said, "Go home! Julie's scan has improved and she does

Portions of this chapter were adapted from *Healing grief: A story of survivorship*, by Joan Heller Miller, EdM (Outskirts Press, 2015).

not need surgery." As part of their healing process from this intense time, Joan and Julie co-authored an inspirational children's book, *My Amazing Hospital Story*.

Our third child, Jeremy, was born in 1992, and he added a big dose of activity, energy, and fun to our family. Our three cheerful kids were great pals and could often be found in the basement, dressed in costumes and acting out plays they took turns co-writing and directing.

Joan

In May of 1999, on the cusp of the new millennium, I was forty-one and on top of life. I had been married to my college sweetheart, Ken, for twenty years. He was a physician specializing in blood disorders and cancer, a tireless profession where he was "on-call" 24/7 with his patients. He was devoted to his calling and, in my opinion, was and still is one of the smartest, most compassionate physicians you can find. His schedule was so grueling that, at times, I'd confess to a couple best friends and family, "In order to get some real attention around here, I probably need to get cancer." Then I'd get pulled back to reality when my mind returned to the harrowing image of the bald women waiting to be seen in Ken's office. I found the clearly sick women frightening, to the point of feeling dread when I visited him during the work day. It was difficult to be a witness to their suffering, but, during those visits, I understood and respected the significance of Ken's desire to serve.

I was in excellent physical health: running, swimming, sleeping well, and eating healthy foods. However, over a six-month period, my body began to feel increasingly unfamiliar. I became more and more fatigued until swimming the length of the pool became harder and harder to do. As I climbed the familiar stairway to the second floor of our house, why did my heartbeat sound like elephants stampeding? Black and blue marks suddenly appeared on my arms and legs, even on my eyelids. I also experienced excruciating pain in my ribs and jaw, as well as a high fever. Why is my body falling apart? What if the doctors can't find a cause, and I have to go on living in pain? What if I never feel like the "old Joan" again? I knew by that point something was not right, but I never considered that I was dying. I was healthy, and happy, and young.

Ken

In October of 1998, Joan developed high fevers, drenching night sweats, a rash, weight loss, and severe rib pain. This went on for ten weeks, during which time we saw an internist, an infectious disease specialist, a rheumatologist, and a neurologist who wondered out loud if Joan had cancer. Joan received a brief course of steroids and then improved. The pain and fevers and wracking cough subsided. Life went "back to normal."

For a brief time, we felt relieved.

Then, four months later, Joan was again bruising easily and became very weak, and I finally asked her to go see her doctor and have blood work done. I called the lab at midnight and they read "white count: 42,000 with blasts; hematocrit, 19; platelets, 40,000." I still remember where I was standing and the cold feeling throughout my chest, mind, and soul as I realized that Joan had leukemia. I sat with this until the morning while trying to grasp, deny, and grieve the fact that Joan was probably going to die and that our three children and I would grow up without her. Our life had just changed forever. I also had this thought: Had I carried this plague home somehow from treating cancer patients and spread it to Joan?

Joan

Ken recommended we go to Johns Hopkins for "further testing." I froze in terror. Me? Stay overnight at a hospital? Call it a phobia if you will, but I was terrified of hospitals. Odd, given my husband's work as a cancer physician, but I had always equated hospitals with death. I never thought it could happen to me. At age seventeen, my dad, a psychiatrist, invited me to accompany him to see a patient in a prison hospital to assess whether he was criminally insane or able to stand trial. Standing a few careful feet behind my dad, a giant of a man who was quite a character, I followed him with trepidation through two massive, locked doors into the prison. As he opened each door, one after the other with a large brass key handed to him by the prison warden, I held my breath as the knot in my stomach tightened. Would someone hurt me? Would I be safe?

Now, twenty years later and with a fresh cancer diagnosis, I faced the entrance of another massive stone structure, Johns Hopkins Oncology Center. Ken dropped me off at the front door of the hospital. "Wait here while I park.

I'll be right back." My mind was racing. I held my breath as the knot in my stomach tightened. Once those elevator doors opened and I got upstairs, I might never get out. I knew this; I felt the truth of this.

Ken returned to find me (after some searching) crouched down, hiding behind an arm chair in the far corner of the hospital lobby, crying wildly, petrified of going upstairs to the torture chamber I envisioned would be waiting for me on the cancer ward.

After this preliminary round of tests, a bone marrow biopsy, and more bloodwork, the doctor came in by the end of the afternoon and gave me the sad news, "You have acute myelogenous leukemia."

Ken

I drove back up to Hopkins late that night to stay with Joan and found her in tears. "I only just turned forty-one years old." I was struggling with the push and pull between the statistics on survival with AML, and the hope that Joan and we as a family would be fortunate and "lucky." It was surreal being with Joan and wondering if this would be the last time we went to Cara's sign language performances, Julie's jazz dance, or Jeremy's basketball games together.

Joan

Will I live or die? Why me? Although knowledge can be a helpful tool, I knew too much from living with an oncologist about all the things that could go wrong and also about my slim chances of survival. The expression on Ken's face and the terror in his eyes communicated this even when words could not. Ken would be all alone, without his partner and friend of twenty-five years. What would he do without me? How would our children, ages five, nine, and fourteen, survive a loss of such great magnitude? Why me?

"You can beat this," my spouse (and medical oncologist) declared. "I will take this journey with you step by step. We'll do this together, for better or for worse." He said this with great tenderness and compassion. I recalled our marriage ceremony twenty years earlier. It was heartbreaking to say goodbye to our three young children and the life I knew and loved to begin Cycle One: my first five weeks of intensive inpatient treatment.

Ken

Once Joan was admitted, transitioning from "Joan" to "the acute leuk in room 260," it felt like the sad movie *Terms of Endearment*, where the audience hopes for a happy ending that doesn't happen. Crucial difference: this was not a movie. Flashing through my mind were memories of meeting Joan, dating, getting married, having three wonderful children, and suddenly facing her death.

The next day I drove the kids, aged then seven, eleven, and fifteen, to the hospital to visit their mother. It was a gloomy visit but the kids tried to keep a brave face. On our way back home, while driving sixty-five miles an hour, we hit a deer bolting across the highway; the animal flew upward and shattered the windshield. I heard all three kids in the backseat screaming and knew that they were alive, although they were covered with broken glass and bits of deer tissue and blood. While Joan was hovering on the edge of life and death at the hospital, we all could have been killed in an instant on the highway.

Following this, I was in a constant state of agitation and stress: trying to be with Joan during the day, with the kids in the evening, and then driving back to the hospital, yet again, to monitor Joan's chemo doses and sleep by her side. Our parents thankfully took turns staying overnight with our kids. It felt lonely in that reclining blue hospital chair. I watched Joan sleep. I watched her breathe, waiting for the next calamity.

Joan

Taking orders and maintaining a level of helpless obedience, nausea and vomiting, loss of my curly hair, of freedom and personal agency began taking its toll. Being awakened throughout the night for important medical observation or to dispense meds, flush out IV lines, and change chemotherapy bags were hospital rules I didn't like, but I understood their importance.

Ken

The next six weeks were terrible beyond words. Joan had multiple central line infections, high-grade fevers and rigors, debilitating bone pain, mouth sores, and an allergic reaction where her jaw and throat swelled. She developed massive painful swelling of her right leg, and she required a walker.

With each episode, there were three different experiences in her hospital room: Joan's pain, my fear, and the medical staff's objective assessment. As an oncologist, I saw so many patients go through this same experience, recover, but then later die. I stopped at the small hospital chapel each day and read, "The Lord is my shepherd, I shall not want."

Joan

Grief began snowballing. With each cumulative traumatic event, healing seemed more impossible physically, spiritually, and psychologically. I could no longer endure further inpatient treatment since I was spiraling into a major depression from the multiple traumatic incidents and unrelentless, unimaginable pain that felt like broken bones. I no longer recognized the person I had become. I had reached a point of terrible despair.

Ken

After five weeks Joan was frail but discharged home; this was exciting and frightening. What was going to happen next? Would an infection steal Joan away, a bleed, or a relapse that would suck away our hope? I was trying to pump joy into our three children's days along with some sense of calm and order, but hope was scant, and calm was scarce.

Getting Joan to go through the additional cycles of chemotherapy was profoundly difficult. She became increasingly angry and belligerent, and I was loving her but hating her behavior at the same time, still praying she'd get through this. Joan became a stranger. She was staying up all night and was angry and aggressive, and this was followed by a deep depression. I pushed and pulled Joan to go through three cycles of consolidation chemotherapy, each followed by one month for recovery. At home, I was accessing her mediport, starting IV fluids and antibiotics, and giving her injections. Instead of a balanced and reciprocating relationship, I felt I needed to be a director, a dictator. My feeling was that if Joan could get through all of her treatments, then she would have the best chance of living out a long life. I went into survival mode for Joan and our entire family; I held to the hope that we could pick up all the emotional pieces at some point if Joan lived. I feared that Joan would suffer from this mania and depression and that both would gobble up all of the time that she and we had left with the children before she died.

The mounting stress was more than I could take. I kept thinking that I would keep things together and then "have the big one," meaning a fatal heart attack, and that would finally put me out of my misery.

Joan

Ken had his established ideas and would not budge. "Joan, you must finish that final round." As a medical oncologist, Ken knew the survival statistics, but he could not actually grasp the mind- body-spirit psychological distress and undiagnosed posttraumatic stress disorder I was experiencing. I felt misunderstood, and I resented feeling forced to continue in this state. I tried to pull myself out of my despair, to be the great mother, great daughter, great wife, but I was physically and mentally drained. I felt miserable, like there was no way out. As my spirit plummeted further into a clinical depression, there was little left I could do by that point aside from curl up in bed with the covers over my head.

Throughout the day, Ken and others tried to persuade me to come out of hiding. I pleaded to them, "Please, let this depression stop; just let me close my eyes and drift off to sleep." My bedroom was my constant place for escape. I kept the blinds drawn; in my dark room, life was quiet.

Depression, for me, was like a curse with physical and psychological torture almost impossible to describe. It felt impossible to have hope that one day the suffering would subside. Depression saturates your entire body, living in every single cell from top to bottom. The physical pain of depression squeezed my brain as if it could explode; pounded like a jackhammer with pain that wouldn't stop. If you've ever been sick with a high fever, your body can go from hot one second to cold the next. You simply aren't yourself anymore; your face is empty with deep circles under your eyes. It felt like hundreds of tiny spiders were crawling madly on every one of my nerve endings. The pain echoed through my body.

Someone must stop this pain. Anything would be better than what I am going through, including death. God, if you really exist, and if you are truly great, why would you let me suffer like this? These thoughts rifled through my brain. Wasn't suffering through cancer treatments enough? My depressed brain kept badgering me: "I'm hurting people I love. This won't get better. My family will be better off without me." No matter how much I tried, I could not decrease the volume. Day after depressed day marched on.

Ken

Our family was struggling with Joan's persistent depression which was like a black hole. I ruminated that Joan was spending her time in remission suffering from a profound depression and not creating memories with the kids. I left the house each day worried that she would take an accidental overdose of pain meds. I hired a companion to sit with her so I could go to work. We saw multiple psychiatrists and psychologists who did not appear to understand our experience—and some were, frankly, quite odd. Joan's depression worsened.

Joan

I'd grown accustomed to Ken's threats: "I can't stand this one more minute. You can't keep doing this to me," as though he experienced the anguish. The tone in his voice was different when he yelled, "Get out of that bed! It is unfair to our children and to me that you keep lying there!" Even in my deep despair, I knew Ken was right. He felt no choice but to have me admitted to a psychiatric unit to help generate a better treatment plan for my intractable depression.

Ken

My loneliness and sense of isolation and helplessness intensified when I could not find a committed psychiatrist. I also experienced increasing isolation from friends and family who didn't know what to do, what to say, or how to help. Joan had two more brief inpatient admissions for depression followed by a lengthier outpatient day program.

Joan

Finally, after days and months of inpatient and outpatient treatment, the right cocktail of medications worked. I found a gifted psychotherapist to help me through the healing process. The "new me" emerged, fortified and richer because of having gone through hell and emerged on the other side.

Ken and Joan

As a couple we learned that loss can be a catalyst for change and an opportunity for personal and interpersonal growth. Individual and couples counseling helped us through our journey and ultimately held the key to transcendence and transformation. We were fortunate. Not only did we go through a cancer diagnosis and treatment (together), but we discovered we could grow through this experience as well.

Joan

Overcoming cancer and the deep depression that followed led me to a new place of insight, and, miraculously, a stronger marriage and a new career that I loved. I grew to love Ken more than ever for helping to save my life and for keeping our family together.

I promised myself that if I somehow survived, I would try to make the road easier and provide hope for children and families facing a similar challenge. Now, as a bereavement counselor working in schools, hospitals, camps, and community mental health settings, I have the privilege of serving children and families facing life-threatening illness or grieving the loss of a loved one.

The hundreds of journal entries I wrote throughout my experiences with cancer and depression became the foundation for my memoir, *Healing Grief, A Story of Survivorship* (Outskirts Press 2015), which I use as a platform to help educate healthcare professionals about the need for psychosocial support and to provide encouragement for families facing cancer or other traumatic loss. Transforming loss into something spiritually richer than before has helped provide me with the answer to "why me?" and has given new meaning to my life.

Ken

Joan's cancer journey and depression left an indelible mark on my psyche. As a parent, I needed to give up the fantasy of providing a "wonderful childhood" for our kids; instead, I grew to understand that overcoming difficult circumstances can translate into raising incredible, resilient adult children. Through Joan's illness I saw her fragility and experienced an anticipated loss. In real terms, however, I also needed to lose and then reshape my self-image because I just couldn't bring forth the consistently positive, caring, and loving self that I wanted to be for Joan, who was my love and my life. Looking back, I appreciate how well I managed with problems that felt beyond my capacity at the time. I also felt even more deeply appreciative of the healing that comes with time, patience, and the dedication of loving friends and family.

Joan and Ken

In the intervening decades, we have weathered a second diagnosis of breast cancer. This June, we will be celebrating our forty-first wedding anniversary. How did we endure? Surviving one life-changing catastrophe after another and then depression ultimately shaped our relationship and outlook on life in a positive way. As a family, we've matured and collectively grown together. We lived through a hurricane together and not only survived, but our bond was strengthened in a way we never expected.

Winston Churchill famously said, "If you're going through hell, keep going." Ken and I were going through hell at the time, and that's just what we did. We had no choice. There were so many times we wanted to stop and give up. But because of our commitment to keep the family together, we refused to give up until we could find a survival plan that would work for both of us. Ultimately, diving directly into the eye of the storm, meeting grief head on, led to a deeper sense of wisdom and healing that we would not have gained otherwise.

Our struggles with loss and survival fueled our desire to make the journey easier for families facing life-threatening illness. Our learning process continues to deepen over time, including the valuable lessons we've learned from others about deep loss and the struggle it takes to survive. We are humbled by their courage and are grateful for this collaborative opportunity.

Time and again, we've discovered that vulnerability and privacy are not opposites. In telling our story, we were initially ashamed to admit the extent of Joan's depression; there remain powerful social stigmas around mental illness. We decided to disclose our full truth because we want others to know that there is life and light and happiness on the other side.

We've learned that the more open and honest we are, the more valuable it is for the listener. It is the telling of the story, warts and all, that deeply connects us as human beings, strengthening and unifying us spiritually as fellow survivors of deep loss who may feel "I thought I was the only one." We hope that, in reading this, people will understand that they are not alone.

How good it feels to know I'm not alone, and that others can understand what I'm going through.

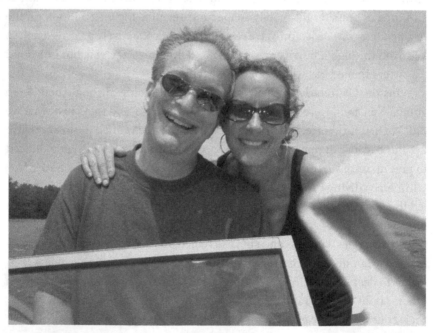

Smooth sailing 20 years beyond leukemia treatment.

About the Authors

Joan Heller Miller, EdM, holds a master's degree in counseling and consulting psychology from Harvard University. She has authored award-winning books and articles for parents and professionals in the field of special education. Over the past twenty years, she has developed bereavement support programs for grieving children and families in schools, camps, and community-based settings and has presented internationally in hospitals, mental health centers, and hospice organizations on psychosocial aspects of cancer care and developing evidence-based coping tools to promote healing and personal growth after a life-threatening illness or death of a loved one. She is the author of the memoir, *Healing Grief: A Story of Survivorship*, by Outskirts Press. Joan brings four unique perspectives to her book: as a two-time survivor of cancer and major depression following treatment, a mental health professional, and the spouse of an oncologist.

Ken Miller, MD, is a medical oncologist and hematologist with more than thirty years of experience. He graduated from Tufts Medical School, trained in internal medicine at Yale, then hematology at the National Institutes of Health and oncology at Johns Hopkins. Dr. Miller was in community practice for fifteen years and then went on to join the faculty at the Yale Cancer Center as the founding Director of the Cancer Survivorship Program. Dr. Miller was then recruited to Dana Farber as the Director of the Lance Armstrong Survivorship Clinic and as a member of the breast cancer program. He later returned with his family to Maryland and was an Associate Professor at the University of Maryland Comprehensive Cancer Center. He is the author of two textbooks on cancer survivorship and one on global cancer care. He has also authored two books on breast cancer, including the recent publication, *The Breast Cancer Book* (Johns Hopkins University Press 2021). Dr. Miller is married to Joan Heller Miller for forty-one years. They are proud parents of three young adults and grandparents of four preschoolers. He and Joan have lectured internationally on the role of empathy in medicine and psychosocial aspects of cancer care for patients and families.

Suggested Resources

Holland, J., & Lewis, S. (2001). *The human side of cancer: Living with hope, coping with uncertainty*. New York: Harper Collins.

Loscalzo, M., Heyison, M., & Butler, R. (2007). *For the women we love: A breast cancer action plan and caregivers guide*. New York: Bartleby Press.

Miller, J. E. H. (2015). *Healing grief: A story of survivorship*. Denver, CO: Outskirts Press.

15

Watching My Wife Move

Joseph V. Simone and Patricia Ann Sheahan Simone

From Joseph V. Simone, MD, to His Dear Wife Pat

This poem is dedicated to Patricia Ann Simone, my wife of fifty-five years, who encouraged me to write and served as my lighthouse to keep me in the right direction.

Watching My Wife Move
Watching her move is thrilling
Not because she is a stunning Hollywood beauty
or publicly sensuous in any obvious way.
But she is so graceful and feminine,
so open, loving and joyful,
that she sparkles.
Is that sparkle in my own eye from seeing her
deeply, her goodness and abundance of love?
Or can this be camouflaged infatuation or lust?

Dare I dissect this fragment of beauty
and risk its destruction?
—Joseph V. Simone (1935–2021)[1]

From Patricia Ann Simone, RN, BA, on the Death of Her Dear Husband Joe

Grief has been like a roller coaster. As Joe's health declined, my emotions were spun on an amusement park thrill ride, but without the amusement or

---

[1] From Joseph V. Simone (2015). *Collected Poems* (p. 20). North Fort Myers, FL: Editorial Rx Press.

the thrill. The endless passes up the steady inclines and down plunging depths took all of my energy. Grief required all of my attention, preventing me from finding some solace in a diversion or distraction. It was always with me. Some days, the feelings took over, climbing to new heights, the pressure tightening against me as the ticking of the track seemed to go on forever, seemingly never reaching the top. With no time to breathe, there I was plummeting down again. The same thoughts wound, over and over, up and down, and round and round. Sometimes it was a persistent worry that spun around. Other times, it was the never-ending paperwork, decisions, and tasks. No starting points or stopping points. The persistent exhaustion.

When Joe died, the roller coaster became more extreme, as if it had joined forces with an unbearable merry-go-round in an insufferable intensity of sadness and exhaustion. As time passed, grief brought new twists and turns. These days, it might even be more like a kiddie ride, but the highs and lows are always there. It comes and goes as it pleases. Throughout all of these phases, two friends have been my constant companions in grief, climbing and spinning with me. They have understood my pain and listened with empathy. Instead of trying to cheer me up or bypass the emotional discomfort, they have acknowledged the sorrow and grief and made room for gratitude and joy. The roller coaster is still there, but they consistently provide comfort, support, and care. I am forever thankful for their friendship.

Well, as always, Joe said it best in his 2015 column in the *Oncology Times*: "This rather lengthy history is a tribute to the best wife, mother, and grandmother I have ever seen in action. And without her rock solid values and support, my life and that of my daughters might have been very different. A strong, unflagging, irrepressible love and her uncompromised values made our family and our marriage what it is. What more can I say? Here we are, married just short of 55 years with a family we can be proud of because of Pat, love, and maybe a small dash of luck."[2].

[2] Simone, Joseph V. (2015, June 10). Pat, love, and luck. Simone's OncOpinion. *Oncology Times* 37(11), 41–42. doi:10.1097/01.COT.0000466853.55875.f4.

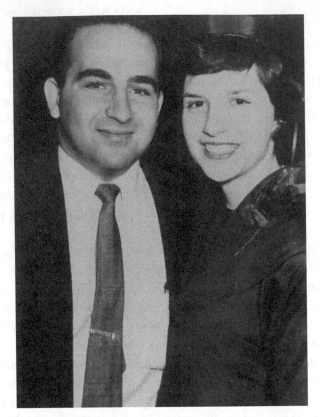

Patricia and Joe Simone circa 1960

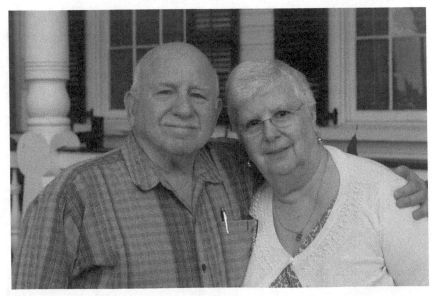

Patricia and Joe Simone 2015

About the Authors

Joseph V. Simone, MD (1935–2021), a pioneering internationally recognized clinical investigator and pediatric oncologist, joined St. Jude's Research Hospital in 1967 and served as Director from 1983 to 1992. He was one of the leaders in finding the first curative treatment for childhood leukemia, and he created both HIV/AIDS and Survivorship clinics for childhood cancer survivors. "Joe," as he was known to all who met him, was a true Renaissance man: clinician-scientist, author, philosopher, poet, and warrior for civil rights. He marched with Martin Luther King, Jr. in Memphis only one week before his tragic assassination. Perhaps as a writer-philosopher, Joe was best known and appreciated for his integrity, columns, and eventual "leadership bible," *Simone's Maxims Updated and Expanded: Understanding Today's Academic Medical Centers* (2012). After leaving St. Jude's, Joe took on leadership roles at cancer centers around the country, including Memorial Sloan-Kettering Cancer Center in New York and the Huntsman Cancer Institute at the University of Utah. Joe was recognized as a 2017 Giant of Cancer Care by the American Society of Clinical Oncology. But to know Joseph V. Simone, MD best is to be aware that he was always, first and foremost, a family man, as we gain a glimpse from the poem *Watching My Wife Move.*

Patricia Ann Sheahan Simone, RN, BA, met her husband, Dr. Joseph Simone, when she was in a registered nurse program. Other than agreeing never to discuss the unmentionable Chicago White Sox versus the Chicago Cubs allegiances with extended family, the rest was a deeply committed sixty years plus love affair. Dr. Simone would never miss the opportunity to refer to Pat as the "Master Mother," foundation for all they accomplished together, personally and professionally.

16

Life Is Loss (... and How I Tolerated It when I Became a House Officer)

A Personal Memoir

Cy A. Stein

When asked to write a chapter for his book, I spent a week pondering how to approach the subject of loss, which I believe is a fundamental property of the human condition, one so basic that all of life could be characterized as the disruption of quotidian existence by a series of losses, some small, others massive. However, all losses require a measure of resolution so that a person may move on to new challenges—and, often enough—new losses.

A few words about my early life: after college at an Ivy League school, I received a PhD from a large, prestigious university. The scientific environment at the time was sizzling, with creative scientific thinking limited only by the imagination of the individual student. I worked hard in the lab and enjoyed it, but I felt the field in which I was working was too limited for my liking. I then made the shift to medicine and medical school, which I greatly enjoyed, mostly because of the friends I made there. The interns and residents I interacted with during my medical school clerkships were a delightful group of men and women who always kept their spirits up despite the relative impoverishment of the hospital in which they worked. But, in the blink of an eye, I was off to internship and residency, naïve about the tsunami that was about to wallop me.

During my earlier life, I was fortunate in not suffering the world-shattering losses so many have had to deal with. Both my parents lived until their later eighties, my grandfathers even longer. One grandmother, with whom I was close, passed when I was six; the other, who lived in California (I grew up in New York), when I was seventeen. While I missed them, I recovered quickly, though I was not highly experienced or sophisticated in managing great personal loss.

It was not until my internship and residency program, at age thirty-two, that I suffered the greatest loss of my life. This involved what I perceived as a complete loss of agency due to my perception of a catastrophic diminution in my status as a valued member of society and my inability to derive much pleasure in life when my days and nights were devoted solely to working and sleeping. My unrelenting schedule and the acute and chronic sleep deprivation caused marital problems and robbed me of any quality time with our new baby. When I express these thoughts to many physicians who are my contemporaries, they are incredulous. "But," many of my flabbergasted contemporaries will insist, "internship and residency were where I learned so much, and where I acquired the technical skills and ways of thinking that allowed me to become a practicing physician. It was an invaluable experience that cannot not be replicated. And if this experience were to be modified in any way, God help us all!"

Any change in the experience meant that fledgling doctors would be missing something undefinable, but vital, to their total experience. Even more, I believe the great fear was that to relieve the pressure on house officers by even a single millimeter of mercury would mean that, with time, the physician product turned out by the residency program would unavoidably deteriorate. That would reflect poorly on anyone in the hospital.

I don't entirely disagree with this reasoning. For a few special trainees, I think internship and residency, even as I experienced it, can be a good way of producing high-quality physicians if administered fairly, as my program was. Many, if not most of the older attending docs who went through this same residency as I did were highly intelligent, pleasant people who seriously desired to help the sick.

Often, as interns and residents we were treated by our elders—meaning the attending physicians—kindly and with respect. With the exception of a few, they understood our physical and emotional struggles, having gone through the same thing themselves, some in the very recent past.

But everyone, attendings and house officers alike, persisted in reasoning from the wrong premise. This was the notion that human beings are automatons that can perform at roughly the same high level with little food or sleep, day in, day out, twenty-four hours a day and more, and under some circumstances almost seven days a week, without a whisper of complaint.

What I was put through in my residency program of nearly forty years ago was appalling. There are 168 hours in a week. We were expected to be working (i.e., in the hospital) for about 100 of them. That means that all other activities—sleeping, eating, showering, pooping, and everything else that counted as living, with no excuses or exceptions—had to be crammed into the other 68. We had one full weekend off when we did not have to appear in the hospital except for Saturday mornings, every three weeks. After working this schedule for a short while, the resulting sleep deprivation became so severe that there was simply no way to "catch up"—as we were, on the basis of no data, informed by the internship directors that we could do on the weekends. (Subsequent research has shown that sleep deprivation cannot be "cured" simply by a good nights' sleep at the end of the week).[1]

How could this insane, dehumanizing schedule not negatively impact my mood, my interactions with loved ones, and my entire view of life, one that narrowed to include only those events that occurred in the hospital? For instance, anything newsworthy happening in the world at large— "fuggedaboudit." The information never penetrated my cerebral cortex, which was too preoccupied with other matters. I was always a "news junkie," but those years are just mist in my memory. Spending time with our new baby, little Allison? Forget about that, too. There just weren't enough hours in the day. I doubted I was of much use to the little girl since I was asleep on my feet half the time and exhausted and irritable the other half. I was living with a sense of chronic unease, knowing there was nothing I could do about it. In retrospect, I see the extent of the loss to my child and myself. But it's hard to know now, and Allison at forty has no recollection of those days. Perhaps that feeling of mine was an extension of the general dehumanization I felt at the time. This was one of the most difficult aspects of residency—that device inside my head, relentlessly tapping out the message that my status in the community had been reduced to that of a serf and that most of my most basic rights as a human being had been abrogated, leaving me like a piñata, swinging in the breeze while someone was taking a shot at me with a bat. And it became very tough to convince myself that this period in my life was time-limited and wasn't my new forever.

Things were even worse the month we worked the ICU. This gig was thirty-six hours on-call, twelve off, with virtually no opportunity to take a break from working or to speak up about anything. Cruel and unusual, for sure. Worse still, absolutely f**king crazy, in my humble opinion. Even now,

---

[1] Choshen-Hillel, S., Ishqer, A., & Mahameed, F., et al. (2021). Acute and chronic sleep deprivation in residents: Cognition and stress biomarkers. *Medical Education* 55, 174–184. https://doi.org/10.1111/medu.14296.

almost forty years later, I still develop a cold sweat thinking about the sleep deprivation imposed on us.

Doctors (myself included) were often so sleep-deprived they couldn't recognize how sleep-deprived they were. After three weeks or so in the ICU, the thought processes of the interns and residents responsible for treating desperately ill patients became so deranged that great ugliness could happen.

For instance, an eighteen-year-old man was admitted with a diagnosis of a urinary tract infection and later decompensated on the floor where I was the junior medical resident. My diagnosis was that he had tricuspid valve insufficiency and right ventricular failure. The cardiac ICU junior resident (a person equal in rank to me), however, refused to accept him to the ICU as a patient and made his feelings about the appropriateness of my diagnosis very clear. I felt his comments were dismissive, devaluating, and, worse, dead wrong. I was certain I was correct and wasn't going to back down. I can behave in a similar way if I think people, especially those in authority, act in a way I consider unjust. From whom did I learn such behavior, which can often be viewed as maladaptive? I think some of it from my mother, who would not tolerate any of her offspring being treated unfairly. The remainder was probably baked in with the cake. It started early. At the age of eight, I observed the consequences of expressing this trait. One day, in summer day camp, I was part of a baseball game for which a very senior counselor had, oh so very carefully, delineated the rules and boundaries. However, when our side came up to bat, this same counselor (Al, whose name I've remembered for the past sixty years) called one of our batters out when he had clearly hit a home run! Oh, for God's sakes, Al, it was clear as day! Enraged, I approached the counselor. "You cheated," I announced right to his face and in a public space. "Son," Al replied. "If you say that again, I'm going to slap you right across the face." Perhaps I believed he didn't really mean it, so I repeated myself: "You cheated," I said again. True to his word, Al slapped me right across my face. It was a painful moment, both physically and emotionally. But at least I had the satisfaction of knowing I was right.

Back to my original story, which occurred during my junior resident year. I diagnosed the cardiac ICU junior resident as sleep-deprived; condition, serious. Several weeks later, after being accepted into the cardiac ICU, the patient left the hospital with a new tricuspid valve. Here was a happy ending for a change, but the same endpoint could have been achieved with far less misery had the cardiac ICU resident been less exhausted and more willing to consider my point of view, think things through, and increase his workload slightly. Nevertheless, I did obtain a measure of satisfaction, an exceedingly rare commodity in those days, from winning the argument with that gentleman who had been so dismissive of my analytical ability, which I still consider to be my strongest suit. The thought of watching this young patient walk out of the hospital under his own power still leaves me with a warm feeling, decades later.

Needless to say, I hated working in the ICU as an intern, and, at my core, there is still a burning anger at how automated and utterly degraded as a human being I felt during those months. This was living for the sake of staying alive, but without any decent quality of life as far as I was concerned. Worse yet, my resident, whom I felt was perpetually scowling and adversarial, was a tough guy to communicate with. How far had I fallen from the professional respect I received during my PhD days and previously!

This is all a great deal for me to admit because, where I come from, one didn't talk about one's deepest feelings with just about—well, *anyone*. Rather, you sucked it up and kept on plugging away, no matter how wretched your existence was. Where the hell did I learn to be different? I don't really know, but if I had to guess, I'd say I got it honestly from both my mother's and father's sides. I'll say no more about the matter of plugging away in misery, other than that some have compared me to a bulldog, in the sense that once I got my teeth into something, I never let go. I think the description is apt, but only when it comes to life goals. In that context, I've found this trait to be enormously helpful, but on occasion it's blinded me to the fact that sometimes I just had to let go, if only for my own sanity. But, back in those days, I had a family that needed to be provided for and that was the number one priority. I did not feel it was possible to simply "let go."

Matters were especially problematic for me because my wife and I had a very difficult baby at home. I wasn't there, didn't spend enough time with them, and couldn't enjoy Allison's developmental milestones, such as crawling, and taking her first steps. My wife felt lonely, especially because all the care of Allison was placed on her shoulders, and very little additional help was available. I was often so exhausted I fell asleep on the couch. My wife felt that she, too, was struggling as she had to provide almost all the child care, manage all the shopping, and handle the payments of all the bills (fortunately, she didn't have to bring in the cash, too). She, too, thought that what the hospital was doing to the house officers was illegal and "disgusting," as she put it years later. After a while, she said, communication between the two of us was virtually cut off because of how the interns were tormented. She said she tried to be sympathetic but it was hard. Forty years on, she still feels the hospital should pay reparations for what they did to us guys and gals. Needless to say, none of this helped our marriage. But, somehow, we stayed together and have been together, at the time of this writing, for forty-five years. If that's not love, what is?

Every problem was worsened by my sleep deprivation. I had trouble finding the right words in which to express myself, and I became intensely irritable and defiant. What do I mean by defiant? It's a truism that if you make someone's life miserable enough, they're going to stop working for you. That was me: I became work-averse. I thought of every way possible to avoid it. If a resident demanded I do something when I was physically exhausted, especially anything difficult or time-consuming, I was always ready with a justification for why it did not need to be done right then. Whatever it was could easily wait until later in the afternoon, or until the next morning, or until just about never. I didn't want to fight with anyone—I wanted to wear my opponents out. Unfortunately, my methods didn't work with those residents much smarter than myself or with those who were truly mean people. That first category included folks who were a pleasure to listen to and the second, thank God, were rare.

My inability to catch up on my sleep deprivation made me a very irritable young man. One night, at 4:15 in the morning, a pharmacist's assistant (PA) arrived at our little call room. My resident and I had been working in the ICU since seven the previous morning and were just about to turn off the light to try to catch some greatly desired sleep. However, the assistant wanted me to make a minor change in a prescription that, under the rules of those days, would have required me to rewrite the entire prescription to be accepted by the pharmacist. But by this time, I was done, finished, and exhausted. The sheer pettiness of the request, coming when it did and from whom, transformed me in an instant from Dr. Jekyll into one nasty badass dude. I was pissed off and in a murderous funk, half asleep but still ready to kill. So, I told that PA where to go (back to the pharmacy) and what to do when he got there (ask the pharmacist to make the correction himself, which is what pharmacists usually did in similar circumstances). Finished and done, and everyone's off to sleep, right? I'm afraid not, for it has been suggested that the author of this piece treated the PA the way he was treated. Perhaps, but I argue by way of exculpation that the PA was near the beginning of a shift, while the author was in the twenty-first hour of his. But, admittedly, I could have done a better job of holding it together.

"Stein," said my resident angrily. "I don't like the way you talk."

What? Was this guy challenging me to a duel instead of trying to get some sleep? I told him that we could discuss anything he wanted to after we both got some shut-eye, all three hours of it that remained before cockcrow. But I knew I had to be careful with this man: my resident was a high-society boy not only with extensive connections to the hospital's Board of Directors, but he also had family members among the other residents. I had no desire for any gossip to also be making rounds. Fortunately for me, after reviewing the matter, the Director of the ICU found nothing amiss with my behavior.

The entire episode left such a sour taste in my mouth I've remembered it for the past four decades. On the one hand, here I was, a thirty-two-year-old man with PhD and MD degrees and a family. On the other, I was being ordered about in the dead of night, exhausted, by an assistant and working with a resident who seemed to be more concerned with the assistant's feelings than with mine. That was the real gut punch: the realization that no matter how hard I worked, and no matter how obedient I was, all my efforts combined were never going to be enough for some of my residents. This was all new to me as I had always been at the top of my class and managed to resolve any intellectual challenges encountered. It all seems so small now, but, at the time, it felt like another body blow to my social status and to my evolving identity as a physician. This is because this small incident combined my sense of loss of social status with my preexisting realization of how vast and complex the practice of medicine is and how impossible it seemed to master, no matter how many years one might train. These feelings were coupled and amplified by my dread of completely screwing things up, which could be worse than dire for another living being. All these thoughts, which I never spoke aloud during internship and residency, led me to the largest loss of personal confidence I've suffered in my life, one that took me several years to work through.

I had already lost my love for medicine: that had been "sweated" out of me during those long nights of sleeplessness. I had also become very disillusioned with many of my fellow house officers, the folks who administered much of the brutality. But I suppose many of them were in survival mode, too, and some may have also been floundering. I don't know anything certain about that; such knowledge was kept secret from all the other house officers, appropriately so.

I'm sure I was no great pleasure to be around in such a sleep-deprived state. But I did my best to "just shut up and do my job" and struggled on a daily, sometimes hourly, basis to convince myself that my resident was always far more intelligent and experienced than I was. Thus, everything I was instructed to do, as I repeated to myself over and over again, represented the best, in fact the optimal, care of the patient. And you know what? It took me several agonizing months, but little by little I was able to brainwash myself to shut up and obey and to persist no matter how fatigued I felt. I would prove to all the doubters (myself included) that I could be that semi-robotic, half-comatose house officer the big boys (there were few big girls in those days) said they wanted. I would make the Faustian bargain and, in selling my soul, ensure my survival in this business. What did that mean in practice? Since I didn't have the neurons for everything, the more creative parts of my being would just have to suffer for now. It was like what Dr. Anthony Fauci (an alumnus of the same program as I, some years previous) alluded to in a recent TV interview. Wow! After thirty-five years I discovered I wasn't alone, that even someone as august as Tony Fauci could admit that during his own internship he would reach down in his distress into the bottom of the tank and find—more distress. Nevertheless, he adjured his listeners, "I somehow sucked it up and plowed through." Note: Fauci and I are both products of New York City, the best place I know for anyone to suffer dire consequences from a bad decision.

There was no way I was going to quit. Despite my own misery, I had a duty to see things through: a duty to my own little family, a duty to my parents, and, finally, a duty to my own ability. I couldn't abandon either group, and especially not my own ability, which has always been my great motivator and often my best friend. Is this pure ego talking? Perhaps so, but that's how I'm put together.

With respect to my sense of duty, I think I come by it naturally. My father once and only once, when I was more than fifty, told me about an incident that commented on his own sense of duty, which I think he passed on to me. During the Second World War, he commanded the anti-aircraft guns aboard a troop transport ship in the South Pacific. More than 500 men were on board. As a Japanese kamikaze fighter, guns blazing, closed on his position at the bow of the ship, at great personal risk he continued to issue orders to the gunners when and where to fire. He refused to abandon the position until the enemy passed over the boat's bow and crashed into the sea. Because he had a safer choice but didn't take it, I consider the course of action my father took that day represented true bravery and the strictest attention to duty at all costs.

Eventually, I realized that I wasn't hired for my intellect (as someone once said to me: "Cy, smart boys and girls are a dime a dozen. It just matters what you produce"), nor my scientific creativity, but to flawlessly perform a detailed, painstakingly difficult job that dealt with constant serious illness and death. How did it feel? Most often, like there was too much weight pressing down on too little shoulder. And when I had that feeling, I couldn't help but remember that I was completely on my own. There was no Human Relations Department to speak with. There was no one to complain to except for a somewhat unsympathetic chief resident, who would tell us residents to "suck it up" and stop being "weak" or something similar. Or, in my case, the same chief resident who told me I had no future as a clinical practitioner after observing me for less than three weeks into my first rotation as an intern. That comment landed like the bite of an asp. Frankly, I was aghast that someone could utter words so impetuous and hurtful to a beginning intern. I lost all respect for the man and fumed about his words for years afterward. As it turned out, and to his credit, he greatly changed his opinion of me as the year progressed. But words can wound, and sometimes you can't take them back, especially if you don't make an effort to do so. It's difficult to describe what the hurt felt like, other than to say—it hurt badly. I think that for a while I felt like the stupidest intern that ever existed, and I continued to feel that way for some time. Nevertheless, while I didn't know how to express myself in the correct jargon, I had a strong sense that my problems were not really related to stupidity but to difficulty in adjusting to my new living circumstances.

A recent veteran of this training program had taught me the following: "Think of your internship and residency this way," he said. "You have just committed a great crime. But you will never be allowed to know what that crime is. Internship and residency are your punishment. Deal with it." Kafka, in his dystopian fantasy, *The Trial*, could not have summed it up better.

Through all this madness and exhaustion, interns and residents were supposed to further educate ourselves by also reading the medical literature in our "spare time"! Difficult to believe, but there were many who did so, including my own addled self. (It was a very competitive group, my internship class. Don't get me wrong . . . there were many fine people who had a place in the program. Sadly, there were also more than a few jerks who were just as work averse as myself but, at the same time, much more willing to dump the work on others. I doubt anyone had complaint of me for behaving in that way!)

But, as I mentioned, to survive, I had to sacrifice a valued part of myself, the creative, inquisitive part. That's what I did, just shut it down. Closed it up. Out of business. "This brain no longer open at this site" or at any other. "Just shut up and do your job" became my mantra. I didn't like it, but it helped get me through the day.

There was one other thing that got me through the day. It was the thought that no matter what they did to me, no matter how miserable, devalued, or otherwise torn to pieces I felt, I would be goddamned if I ever pulled this crap on anyone else, ever. Therefore, I swore a mighty oath to myself alone that I would treat my interns with dignity and that I would try to express to them the notion that we are all in this together. I don't know if my strategy worked because there was no formal evaluation of the residents by their interns. But I overheard a bunch of guys informally rating their residents about three-quarters of the way through their intern year. It was the time when the first crocuses appeared. The very late winter and early spring was a beautiful time of year because the flowering crocuses meant the ordeal was almost over for everyone. And I was very glad to hear what the interns said about me. Of course, when I was working with my own interns, it was rarely at four in the morning, when, frankly, I was not at my best. Rather, as a resident, I dealt with my interns most often in the full light of day, when I was better rested.

Otherwise, during those years (1982–1984), the psychic burden on me was enormous. I felt like a newly disempowered marionette whom anyone could abuse *ad libitum*. I had inexplicably and through no fault of my own been wrenched out of the comfortable life I knew well into a strange, frightening, bizarro society where the rules were different and where I, despite all I'd already accomplished, was a member of its lowest social stratum.

Every illusion I ever had about patient care was torn up and tossed out, much like an old wet carpet after a flood. I became angry at the senior physicians who set up this training program and had allowed it to continue unchanged, year after year. And at some level, though I'm ashamed to admit it, I think I became a little angry at the patients, too. Weren't they the ones denying me the sleep I so craved, and why didn't they stop it? And how could I ever think of being a doctor if I was angry toward patients? These thoughts greatly troubled me, but, thank goodness, the conflicting feelings about patient care dissipated soon after I graduated the residency program.

Despite the value of having received training in such a prestigious program, despite however much I, as a fledgling doctor, learned (granted, it was an enormous amount), I had to ask myself if it was worth the years of sleep deprivation and other abuses. I had to seriously wonder if there weren't a better way of imparting the lessons we had to learn, other than by causing the learners such misery. I had to ask if the lesson I learned—that when on call late at night, cut every corner possible to ensure you got some sleep—was the right lesson to learn. Or, if you did call for help in the middle of the night that you were somehow "weak," so think carefully before doing so. I was saddened by the thought of those kind little comments everyone needs once in a while to keep going but that I never heard from my residents—words such as "I'm sorry," or "I was rude and made a mistake," or "You did a good job." Now, gazing back through the decades with some objectivity, I can see that many of my residents were also sleep-deprived, though if confronted they either would have denied it or instead insist it truly didn't affect their performance in any way that affected the quality of patient care.

Sadly, their behavior only recapitulated the behavior of those who trained *them*. As I mentioned before, I did my best to eschew such behavior because not doing so would violate my own personal prime directive. As in the simple, lucid words written in the Hebrew scriptures millennia ago by the prophet Micah, we, all of us, must always refrain from doing injustice.

With my stomach in a perpetual knot even after taking the appropriate medicine and a case of what surely resembled posttraumatic stress disorder, I left the hospital after successfully graduating from the program.

How did I handle the three years of internship and residency? Poorly, I suppose. I badly needed time off, but I had a young family and had to make a living for all of us. That meant I had no choice but to do my duty to my family and to myself and plow through the system, protecting myself as best as I could and ensuring that I never, ever behaved in the same way to others as they behaved to me. But I still lived in a very dark place, as if I had a chip on my shoulder, waiting for a fight.

And then, on the evening of March 3–4, 1984, a patient walked into the Emergency Room at my hospital with a complaint of a fever and an earache. That night, there were two junior residents on call at the hospital. I was the junior resident that poor, sick teenage girl was *not* assigned to when she arrived on the floor. By the early morning, the patient had died. After that sad and terrible event, years of media interest, wild accusations, courtroom drama, and the Bell Commission Report, interns and residents would never be treated the same again. This awful patient outcome finally woke up the medical training system and resulted in significant work hour rules to prevent exhaustion and poor patient outcomes.

That was years in the future. At the time, I was off to my fellowship in another very prestigious institution. But who exactly was I now, and could I cope with some of the same types of stresses and pressures that had brought me to the brink as an intern and resident?

Fortunately, my third year in the residency program played a major role in restoring my sanity. The schedule wasn't so crazy, and I had more time to myself and to spend with the family. The feeling of falling out of love with medicine dissipated. I had also come to know one of the clinician-scientists who attended patients for part of his workweek but otherwise holed himself up in his lab the rest of the time. I had the option of spending six months in his lab or instead doing another six months of patient care. At that time in my life, the option of taking some time away from patient care to be in the lab seemed especially appealing.

I worked for my new mentor for six months and enjoyed my laboratory experience, though, frankly, I don't remember much of it. This was probably because there were no conflicts among the others in the lab and no existential problems emerging to threaten the boss, who was steady, stable, and predictable. It was during that year that I had time to reflect on the experience of being a house officer and on the practice of medicine in general. It was then that I came to the irrevocable decision that the full-time practice of medicine was not for me. However, the notion that I would abandon patient care completely was also not going to happen. While I was determined not to be reduced to a one-patient-every-twenty-minutes physician, I realized that attending patients had become a very important part of my life— provided I wasn't sleep-deprived. I never appreciated patient care more than in that third year of residency, and, strangely, I never appreciated science more either. Thus, this became the career I pursued, or persevered with (or perseverated in, as some might say) for the past thirty-five years. I would be a clinician-scientist, much the way my mentor in that third year was, incorporating the best of both worlds into my own career. Of course, there were other factors that helped me arrive at this life-altering, fateful decision, but, at the time, this seemed to be the only way forward for me. And I held to this concept, this plan of mine, for many years, despite efforts—some well-intentioned, others not so much so—to persuade me to give it up, until my retirement in 2020, the year of the pandemic, when so very many things changed.

Finally, a simple question has been posed to me: How did I, who disliked the system as I experienced it, manage to not only recover from its abuses but to thrive in it? Part of the answer is that I accepted the system for what it was and managed to make myself very useful when my expertise as a scientist came to be valued during my fellowship. (However, it has never been possible to recover all of that sense of confidence I had in my naïve days before internship.) During my fellowship, I discovered an area of biomedical research that was important yet underdeveloped. Falling in love with the subject, I worked on it assiduously as an assistant professor, as if this small area of interest was, with the exception of my family, the most important subject of interest on the entire planet. It was a labor of love. Several years later, I was asked to review the area for *Science*, one of the most prestigious and well-respected peer-reviewed journals. The paper I produced put me on the international map, launched my scientific career, and helped keep me in orbit for decades.

About the Author

Cy A. Stein, MD, PhD, is an internationally renowned pioneer in the field of oligonucleotide therapeutics. He received his PhD in chemistry at Stanford University under the mentorship of Henry Taube, FRSC, the 1983 Nobel Prize winner in Chemistry. Dr. Stein's thesis work is still taught to graduate students at Caltech as "classic." Dr. Stein went on to receive his MD at the Albert Einstein College of Medicine. He has held Professorships of Medicine and Molecular Pharmacology at Albert Einstein and Columbia University. He has also served as Attending Physician and Director of Medical Genitourinary Pharmacology at Montefiore Medical Center and the Chair of Medical Oncology at City of Hope National Medical Center. Dr. Stein co-founded the Oligonucleotide Therapeutics Society and was an editor of the journal *Oligonucleotides* for twenty-one years. In addition to his extraordinary research and leadership achievements, Dr. Stein has maintained a prominent prostate cancer practice. He retired in 2021 and embarked on his second vocation as a writer of historical fiction. His latest work, *Caligula and I*, the second volume in the Vox Populi Series (the first is *The Medicus Codex*) was selected by Kirkus Reviews as one of the top 100 Indie books of 2021.

17

Mourning and Restoration

Craig D. Blinderman

Come, come, whoever you are,
wanderer, worshiper, lover of leaving,
it doesn't matter.
Ours is not a caravan of despair.
Come, even if you have broken your vow a hundred times.
Come, come again, come.

—Jelaluddin Rumi (1207–1273)

The snow of yesterday
That fell like cherry blossoms
Is water once again

—Gozan (1789)

In the early days of September 2020, while quarantining on a distant Hawaiian island, my gaze came to rest on a red-crested cardinal. As the Pacific light shrouded the plumeria tree and the silky flowers glowed in the morning sun, I noticed their unique song. Or was it the song that manifested the cardinal? I couldn't tell. I was simply a listening subject, gazing at the sky and resting "in the grace of the world," as Wendell Berry describes this splendor of immediacy, where the innumerable expressions of the world hold us and sorrow dissipates. And then, as if awakening from a fugue, the following question bubbled up and I immediately began to write: "What must we do before the matter ends and life returns to its vastness?"

"Behold the songbird," a voice seemed to answer.

I was in New York City on September 11, 2001. I was completing my sub-internship as a medical student at Columbia's Allen Pavilion Hospital, located in the Northern Manhattan neighborhood of Inwood. I was on call that day, covering the emergency department's admissions for the general medical service I was assigned to. The morning news revealed what we could see with our own eyes since we could view the Twin Towers downtown from our Inwood perch. Sitting in a large room with southern-facing windows, we were trying to discuss our patients until my senior resident abruptly exclaimed, "I don't see them anymore!"

The billowing clouds of gray smoke gave way to nothingness. The buildings had crumbled, disappeared. I remember not being so much paralyzed with shock but struck by something familiar—this was a terrorist attack. I was filled with the gravity of what that meant and the dread and trauma—individually and collectively—it would cause. I had been in Israel for medical school during much of the Second Intifada, witnessing the first-hand news reporting and unfiltered grieving that accompanied each bombing and the impact it had on Israelis and others. I remember the local bus station in Beer Sheva was the source of an attack, and our medical school went into a kind of lockdown. I recall being on call for the trauma surgery team when the Israeli Defense Forces (IDF) evacuated a young Palestinian from Gaza who had un-successfully detonated a bomb and was nearly killed in the process, and the attention he received from the Israeli surgical team. Somehow the care he received seemed to suggest that every life mattered, any loss of life can be grieved and therefore is worth saving.

There was a way in which these attacks became woven into everyday life, perhaps like mass shootings in the United States, as a consequence of the status quo, and integrated into what society tolerates. In a strange and sad way, I had become used to the occurrence, accepted its reality. However, the attack on September 11 was something else and on a scale not seen before. As we were forced to simultaneously take in this moment in history, residents and hospital teams were expected to stick to one directive that day: discharge as many individuals as possible to make way for the influx of patients we expected to be transferred from downtown hospitals because they would experience a surge in disaster-related traumas and injuries filling their emergency departments and medical wards. But the Allen Pavilion's emergency room was astonishingly quiet. There was no mass transfer of patients from downtown hospitals. No survivors needing emergency treatment. I sat in the Emergency Department in our northern corner of Manhattan feeling bored, useless, isolated from what was happening below 14th Street. It was an eerily quiet evening. Not even local residents sought care that night. Perhaps it is what I needed—a moment of reflection. It was too late for anything else.

And somehow the terrible and unfathomable cleared the way for something remarkable—collective empathy. The following day, September 12, 2001, was perhaps the most peaceful day in New York City's history. Its denizens, in the wake of this unimaginable destruction and trauma, displayed a palpable kindness and recognition of our interconnectedness. Walking down 24th Street in Chelsea, I noticed more eyes making contact. We were looking at each other. Neighbors saw neighbors, perhaps for the first time. It was as if we were saying to each other with our glances: "We are all in this thing together."

This empathic potential still resides in the city, like the cathode of a battery, waiting to connect with the anode of loss and sorrow, releasing kindness. Some part of me was already preparing myself to behold the songbird. To be with what is.

During the endless days of March and April 2020, New York City experienced more than 20,000 COVID-19 deaths and was considered the "epicenter" of a new global pandemic. Ambulance sirens were heard all day and night. Protective equipment was in short supply. Nursing homes witnessed the virus's contagion at staggering rates, with elderly and debilitated patients coming in by the dozens, gasping for breath, scared they would die and never see their loved ones again. Our hospital and our lives were quickly transformed. Clinics would now operate remotely via telehealth, chemotherapy appointments were cancelled and put on hold indefinitely, there were no further elective surgeries. Initially, I tried to help train our outpatient providers to communicate with their most vulnerable patients, addressing their goals of care should they become sick from this new virus. I helped adapt and draft scripts to be used for clinicians not familiar with advance care planning conversations and then trained them to take on this role. I witnessed surgeons and outpatient providers be redeployed to provide critical care services or work in the COVID screening tent. Endoscopy suite and cardiac interventional teams were mobilized to inpatient settings to manage ventilators and other tasks. Anesthesiologists became part of a new family liaison team for critically ill patients.[1] We were all too aware of the risks of contagion at this uncertain time after seeing the nightmare images from hospitals in Bergamo, Italy. We were all afraid. Who should come into the hospital? Who was "essential"? Would we have enough PPE? Would I carry

---

[1] Periyakoil, V. J., Blinderman, C. D., & Schechter, W. S. (2020). Longitudinal coaching and decision support provided by a patient-family liaison promotes goal-concordant care. *Journal of the American Geriatric Society 68*(9), 1933–1935.

this new virus on my clothing back to my partner? Would I be able to see and hug my daughter? What were the risks for me personally? Did we sign up for this emergency frontline force when we went to medical school?

I spent most of my clinical effort during those months running a new eight-bed hospice unit in our hospital.[2] Overnight, walls were erected and two negative pressure rooms were created in an unused, post-acute care unit (PACU) extension. It was a part of the hospital I would have never visited. The unit was necessary, and, as the director of palliative care, I was asked to oversee it. We had never had a hospice unit in our hospital, so this was a completely new experience and intervention. I was given a small staff of oncology nurses, physician assistants, and a hospice liaison nurse. What would the suffering look like? How much different would it be from other patients at the end of life? Would there be more challenges in managing their symptoms? Their secretions and shortness of breath? Their delirium?

Despite the uncertainty and new responsibility, I think some part of me was grateful that this is where I would largely provide clinical care. In a hospice unit, things would inevitably be slowed down, and there were after all, only eight beds, so it felt manageable. I could focus my attention on making sure this operation went well as possible while at the same time coordinating a number of other palliative care efforts across the medical campus and the larger hospital institution.[3] We didn't know what degree of symptoms and pain might emerge with this deadly virus in patients not receiving life support. I felt that I would be most useful in this task to make sure it was managed well and to inform others immediately on any unexpected challenges. My gratitude increased as I saw the faces of some of my colleagues, holding back tears, a state of half-dazed panic and grief, a mix of duty and exhaustion. I felt guilty. Like maybe I needed to do more. My dose of clinical effort was in the form of a tolerable infusion on the hospice unit, not the massive boluses received in the emergency department, critical care units, and medicine wards. At the same time, I was also trying to manage my outpatients through new telehealth portals. There never seemed like there was enough time in the day. And yet I was grateful to be part of it all. To be at this institution, at this

[2] https://www.npr.org/2020/05/24/861630528/new-york-doctor-shares-inside-look-at-caring-for-end-of-life-covid-19-patients.
[3] Blinderman, C. D., Adelman, R., Kumaraiah, D., Pan, C. X., Palathra, B. C., Kaley, K., Trongone, N., & Spillane, K. (2021). A comprehensive approach to palliative care during the coronavirus pandemic. *Journal of Palliative Medicine 24*(7), 1017–1022.

time, in this moment. Gratitude that I could contribute when there was so much at stake. I felt valued and fortunate.

Once the hospice unit became a reality, I vowed to create a refuge from the chaos all around us. I vowed to provide slow and methodical care to the dying and their families. We would start our day with a short meditation—myself, the nurses and our physician assistant staff, and, when possible, our fellow. We allowed a word or feeling to be our intention for the day. Allowing this to be like a bath for us, a little bit of medicine, before we crossed the threshold. I asked our Buddhist chaplain for ideas. How can we transform this "pop up" hospice unit into a place to honor and care for the dying? He suggested covering it with Tibetan mandalas. And so we did. Allowing myself to feel that we were guiding ourselves and the dying into the unknown. On the other side of the wall would be the negative pressure rooms that would contain dying individuals who, only a few weeks ago, both they and their loved ones would never have imagined that this would be their fate. We were near a bridge and large floor-to-ceiling windows provided a perspective of expansiveness even as we felt isolated. It would be a safe haven for staff and patients alike.

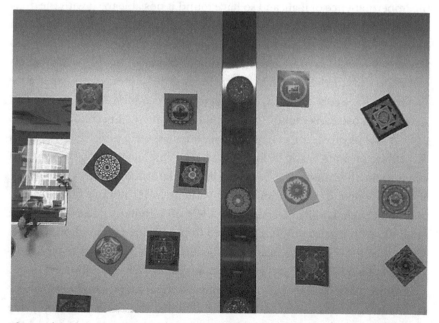

Photo of the hospice unit wall at the Columbia University Irving Medical Center/New York-Presbyterian Hospital. April 2020.

I have always felt more at home in medicine when patients were at the end of their lives. Like many of us, my first intimate encounter with dying was when my grandfather was at the end of his life, dying of heart failure at then Roosevelt Hospital in Manhattan. I recall his isolation, his fear, his loss of hope. I don't think the doctors were really explaining or preparing him for what would be happening next—his death. I would visit him after my classes at Columbia, as a philosophy graduate student, before I knew anything about medicine. In some ways, this experience of seeing the lack of attention to his suffering at the end of life was like a seed planted in me. In medical school, this seed sprouted into a tree. Nourished with my own philosophical and religious readings, from Richard Rorty to Bahá'u'lláh and Krishnamurti, I was inclined to explore how medicine and its practitioners approach suffering, time, personal identity, meaning, and death. During my internal medicine rotation in Jerusalem, I had the opportunity to learn about palliative care from one of the international leaders in the field, Nathan Cherny. I recognized clearly that this field of medicine was not only interested in these philosophical and spiritual intersections with serious illness, but its core—being with uncertainty and impermanence—was familiar terrain for me. In my meditation practice, I learned to appreciate the fleeting, transient nature of things, the impermanence of it all, and so have found it possible to sit with the difficulties as they arise, both within myself and my patients. I learned that I am most at ease and capable in medicine when I am evaluating and attending to the immediate discomfort and distressing concerns of my patients. This attention to suffering is what was missing in my grandfather's dying experience and what I have committed in my professional life to improving.

During those early months of the pandemic, many of us felt like we were not capable of providing enough—or perhaps we were providing too much out of fear and the desire to fight off death. What do we even recommend when so much is unknown? With our limited knowledge, could we give adequate prognostic information to our patients in respiratory failure, guide them and their families according to their underlying values? Were some families given a grim prognosis and led to pursue care focused on comfort rather than life-sustaining treatments, believing they would never survive?

This was a new virus and there were many unanswered questions.

In those early days, we saw a disproportionate number of people of color dying on our hospice unit. At first, I assumed that this result was simply due to the demographics of the neighborhood—Washington Heights—and the local nursing homes that were hit so hard by the virus. I reasoned that this disparity was what we should expect to see. But later, when reports became available not only in NYC but nationwide that this disparity was everywhere, I felt a sense of shame and discomfort. The idea of justice in healthcare always loomed large for me. I recall in Israel the disparities in care that Bedouin families received compared with Jewish Israelis. Though their healthcare outcomes were much better than in neighboring Arab countries, it nonetheless revealed how systems can create disparities even as they actively pursue policies and practices to best care for the least well off. A Rawlsian notion of justice is baked into how I see the world when it comes to healthcare policy. On our hospice unit, most of our patients—more than 70%[4]—were Black and LatinX men and women and one Black transgender woman.

I comforted myself with the belief that our hospice unit would provide a more peaceful end to their lives than the one that was *almost inevitable*— being sedated on a ventilator, condemned to never see their loved ones again. At least on the hospice unit we allowed families to visit. We created the space for loved ones to say goodbye, to touch and hold their dying parent, spouse, brother, and sister. We were told over and over again how much this was a blessing. Families were able to see with their own eyes the deadly consequences of this virus. This seemed to allow for greater acceptance and gratitude that they at least had an easier death. Later, as we received more patients transferred from the ICU, some of whom spent weeks or months receiving intensive care, their families were relieved to finally see their loved ones after enduring painful weeks of separation, medical updates, uncertainty, and FaceTime coordinated visits.

Ocean Vuong writes, "Isn't that the saddest thing in the world, Ma? A comma forced to be a period?" These lives had more commas, but a deadly virus turned them into periods. And all those periods seemed to bleed together into gray. Like the gray clouds that inhabited Manhattan for much of March and April, it also creeped into the hospital rooms and the spaces we inhabited. We worked in that gray area. Our patients seemed gray. The sheer number of deaths on the hospice unit—sometimes three or four in a day— was hard to fathom. I felt myself becoming numb. Fearing that gray bodies were all that there was.

Until Jamie.

---

[4] Sun, H., Lee, J., Meyer, B. J., Myers, E. L., Nishikawa, M. S., Tischler, J. L., & Blinderman, C.D. (2020). Characteristics and palliative care needs of COVID-19 patients receiving comfort-directed care. *Journal of the American Geriatric Society 68*(6), 1162–1164.

Jamie was our one transgender patient on the hospice unit. Unlike the others, I knew her, having cared for her a few months prior.

She taught me what I, and all of us, had truly lost.

Jamie (not her real name) was a fifty-nine-year-old Black male-to-female transgender homeless woman. She was the youngest of five children but was estranged from all her living family members. She had been living in the NYC shelter system for more than forty years and had previously been incarcerated. Her color, gender, and undomiciled status meant she was extremely likely to suffer poor health or be killed. She had been diagnosed with an aggressive squamous cell carcinoma six months prior to my meeting her. She underwent chemotherapy, radiation therapy, and surgery, including a diverting colectomy, leaving her with a permanent ostomy. She had several other medical problems—chronic kidney disease, heart disease, diabetes, major depression, and chronic lymphedema. I had first met her during a hospital admission for rectal bleeding and intractable pain. She was disheveled, short-tempered, and often in distress. She complained that she wasn't being listened to. She was noted to have inconsistent oncology follow-up despite staff visiting her at the homeless shelter across the street and attempting to take her to medical appointments.

Psychiatry had been consulted because of "treatment-interfering behaviors" and to evaluate her capacity to refuse medical interventions. Per collateral information from the medical team, Jamie had been intermittently disruptive of her care and of the environment on the unit. That said, she had not engaged in any behaviors that could be characterized as dangerous, paranoid, or psychotic. The psychiatrist suspected long-standing maladaptive personality traits, poor coping, and limited distress tolerance.

During that admission, I remember having multiple conversations with her about her pain and how her behaviors were likely related to, or at least exacerbated by, poorly managed pain. We started a patient-controlled analgesia (PCA) device and provided extensive education to help optimize her pain management. Within a few days she was much more comfortable. I noticed that when her pain was better controlled, she displayed more kind gestures ("I should call him"), generosity ("they can just have all my stuff"), and humor ("that's nothing, you should have seen me when I was . . . "). I rotated off service at the end of the week, and our team continued to follow her during her hospitalization and helped clarify her goals of care, optimized her pain regimen, and coordinated care with her other providers. I had hoped we would see her in our outpatient palliative care clinic. And then the coronavirus pandemic hit NYC.

Jamie was arguably the most vulnerable and marginalized individual I had cared for. Something about her wanted me to save her. I felt a strange connection. Our family origins and circumstances of birth couldn't be more different. I cannot begin to understand the impact that discrimination and racism has had on her life given the color of her skin and a body and gender incongruent with her identity. Intolerance manifests as the delusion of separateness—"you are not me"—and all the pain that can create. I remember as a four- or five-year old boy watching a cross burning on my lawn in my childhood suburban home on Long Island. Many years later I can still feel the shame and horror of that night. It left in me a feeling of displacement and rejection. We literally moved out of that neighborhood to another town, another school district. Would this early act of hate—against something I had no control over—be a source of my affinity for the vulnerable, displaced, and discriminated against? I wanted to save Jamie from the cruel fate of her life and the degrading systems she was subject to. Sometimes you just look out at the world, and it seems all too much. And you find yourself saying, "Not this person. No, you will not do that to *this* person."

Taking care of Jamie in her last days of life was agonizing. I knew that we had failed her and so many others like her because of racist, economic, and class structures deeply entrenched in our healthcare and public social service systems. I lost whatever faith I had that we could truly save people. I felt that, at a minimum, we should be able to take better care of the least well-off, the most vulnerable, the ones whom our public health colleagues taught us are those at highest risk of morbidity and death. I was ashamed and disheartened that high-quality healthcare was so elusive for so many and for a predictable population—Black, indigenous people, people of color, and the LGBQT+ communities. I felt distraught that the previous efforts we had made—to bring her to her appointments and try to coordinate social services, for example—were for naught. Her vulnerability and status left her more likely to become infected and to die from this new virus.

Perhaps I had always known that our healthcare system had major failings. I had been a long-time critic of the medical-industrial complex. I had seen how misguided forces, more concerned with profit than providing care, held a tight grip over the systems we worked in. But this time, I felt a degree of impotence, guilt, and shame that was difficult to recover from. The ugly truth was hemorrhaging out of whatever patchwork gauze and stitches I had applied to my mind to allow me to believe that our system could help the most vulnerable.

I had looked forward to seeing Jamie in my outpatient clinic. I imagined bearing witness to her story—her life on the streets of NYC, her drug use, her estrangement from her family, her time in prison, her journey to understand her own identity What and who did she care for? Where and with whom would she feel safe? What goals and aspirations did she have?

I never got to ask any of these questions. And so it felt like a kind of abandonment. That I had cared for someone without fully exploring what mattered most. The failure was mine alone.

On our hospice unit, I watched her atrophied muscles become weaker until she could no longer lift her arms. Her belly was bloated and tender. Her eyes half open. Her consciousness diminishing more and more each day. I aggressively titrated her opioid infusion. I could not bear the thought that after a life of so much pain and so much injustice that she would die with any discomfort whatsoever.

There was no chance she would recover. I accepted that now. She was approaching the end of her life, and I vowed silently under my N95 mask that she would not suffer any more. I made sure she was deeply sedated. And, as her sedation increased and death was approaching, I realized how much we had lost. The possibility to have spent more time getting to know Jamie. To explore her world and navigate the challenges of her health and condition together. This is the privilege of the doctor–patient relationship: *to be in relationship*. And this seemed no longer possible, at least not in the conventional sense, as there would be no additional time to develop a relationship. I started to awaken to the reality that loss is the defining quality of our lives. We hope that the future will continue and that we will be able to have another opportunity. But opportunities are lost.

Judith Butler writes, "[I]n this world, as we know, lives are not equally valued; their claim against being injured or killed is not always registered. And one reason for this is that their lives are not considered worthy of grief, or grievable." She goes on to write, "The reasons for this are many, and they include racism, xenophobia, homophobia and transphobia, misogyny, and the systemic disregard for the poor and dispossessed. We live, in a daily way, with knowledge of nameless groups of people abandoned to death, on the borders of countries with closed borders, in the Mediterranean Sea, in countries where poverty and lack of access to food and health care has become overwhelming."[5]

---

[5] Butler, J. (2020). *The force of non-violence* (p. 28). London: Verso.

This was a crushing moral diagnosis of our world: that some lives are more valued than others. This analysis was speaking to me when I was at the peak of my distress in caring for patients dying of COVID-19. I was reading Butler at that time. I knew she was right. And that made me even more distraught. But she also offered hope. Hope in imagining a world that we would want to live in. A world where state-sanctioned violence and systemic injustices are not tolerated. A world where we allow the precarity of our existence and our interdependency to inform our morality and our politics. A world where lives are valued and protected. A world that truly mourned the loss of every life.

In caring for Jamie on the hospice unit, I was struck not only by Butler's words and the possibility of Jamie's life not being considered "grievable," but by the preciousness of the familiar. Previously, patients on the hospice unit seemed anonymous. They came to life only through their relationships with their closest relatives, a fraction of their totality. But with Jamie there had been an experience of her as a person and the beginning of a relationship, based on trust and beneficence. This *particular* person felt precious to me. Precious in that familiar way when we come across a friend we haven't seen in a while, and we notice them stand out in a crowd.

At this time, in April 2020, I began sewing a *rakasu*—a traditional Zen practitioner's garment, worn around the neck, like a bib. This was part of a tradition in becoming a formal Zen student. The *rakasu* was thought to orig-inate in China, as a miniature *Kāṣāya*, a monk's formal robe, when Buddhists were persecuted for wearing such robes. The process of sewing a *rakasu*, met-aphorically and in some way quite literally, is that you are sewing your life into the fabric that is to be worn by the practitioner after taking their vows. It may even symbolize the "vast robe of liberation" that connects all of us. It is the unique expression of the practitioner, which itself is an expression of the universal. I had sewn Jamie into the *rakasu*, into my own vows to benefit all beings. I vowed to remember her and to let her life and struggle be part of my thoughts and actions for the benefit of others.

Behold the songbird, its precarity and preciousness.

I never missed the 7 P.M. cheers for frontline workers. No matter how busy I was, I always made certain to be home before they began, or at least step out of the hospital to witness the city's catharsis.[6] I would bang my pot or the rain-water drainage pipe on my terrace wall like it was a *mokugyo*—the wooden

---

[6] https://www.newyorker.com/podcast/the-new-yorker-radio-hour/amid-a-pandemic-catharsis-at-seven-oclock.

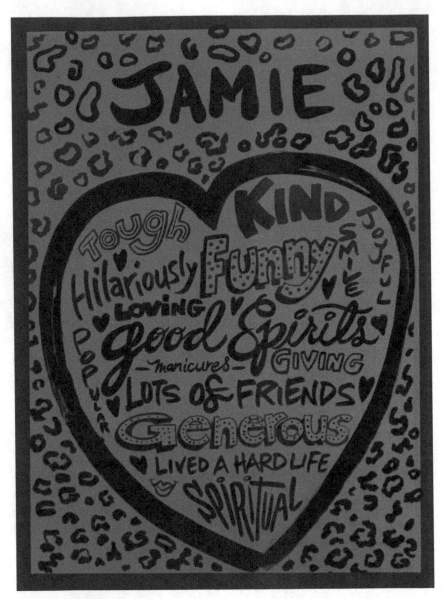

"Jamie's" poster

Source: Artwork by Soren Glassing

fish drum used in Zen monasteries. I imagined that we were all chanting the unsurpassable mantra that clears all pain, The Heart Sutra, or "The Heart of the Perfection of Wisdom" (in Sanskrit *Prajñāpāramitāhṛdaya*). I wanted this "Heart Sutra" of our 7 P.M. catharsis to resonate beyond my neighbors' ears, to include the buildings themselves, the trees, the birds, and all beings in need of compassion. In the same way that September 12 revealed the swell of kindness and interconnectedness after tragedy, the 7 P.M. cheering was our moment of collective empathy. The clapping, horns, banging pots and pans, and every conceivable noise you could imagine brought me to tears. It gave me hope and recharged my depleted batteries each day.

But it was also a moral calling. That we can be better. That we can cheer for decency. We can cheer for Black lives. We can cheer for the holy. We can cheer for our heroes. We can cheer for ourselves. We can let the cacophony remind us of all that we have lost and all that we hoped to improve.

Eight months after opening the hospice unit, when the 7 P.M. cheers had faded, after a deadly summer of civil disquiet, protests, and a raging pandemic, I sought refuge on a distant island in the Pacific. As it happened, one morning I allowed a songbird to fill my brokenness and remind me what we must do before the matter ends and life returns to its vastness. The words "Behold the songbird" became "Behold the world." That is to say, include and bear witness to everything.

But how do we create space to hold those things we don't agree with or prefer not to have happened? How do we allow for that space to open—where words are not permitted, where we can both grieve and take responsibility for all that has been and restore what has been broken?

This is the incomprehensible space between mourning and restoration.

About the Author

Craig D. Blinderman, MD, is a palliative medicine physician in New York. He is Director of the Adult Palliative Care Service at Columbia University Irving Medical Center/New York-Presbyterian Hospital and Program Director of the Hospice and Palliative Medicine Fellowship at New York-Presbyterian Hospital. His academic and personal interests are at the intersection of medicine, ethics, literature, philosophy, and Zen practice. His publications have ranged from early palliative care in lung cancer patients to cancer pain management and existential distress. He is currently the section editor for case discussions in the *Journal of Palliative Medicine*. His teaching focuses on decision-making at the end of life, the role of palliative care in global health, medical ethics, and bringing contemplative care practices to the bedside. He also has a strong interest in teaching and developing programs to improve students' and residents' skills in communication and care for the dying. He serves on the advisory board for the New York Zen Center for Contemplative Care.

Suggested Resources

Berry, W. (2009). *The selected poems of Wendell Berry*. Berkeley: Counterpoint.

Butler, J. (2020). *The force of nonviolence: The ethical in the political*. London: Verso.

Krishnamurti, J. (1984). *On love and loneliness*. San Francisco: HarperOne.

Shunryu Suzuki. (1970). *Zen mind, beginner's mind: Informal talks on Zen meditation and practice*. New York: Weatherhill.

"Va, pensiero, sull'ali dorate." (2001). From Giuseppe Verdi's opera *Nabucco* performed by the Metropolitan Opera Chorus. https://www.metopera.org/discover/video/?videoName=nabucco-va-pensiero&videoId=808137918001.

Conclusion

Loss

We Can Do Better

Matthew Loscalzo, Marshall Forstein, and Linda A. Klein

Loss Defined

In many ways, as described in the Introduction, the three years of writing *Loss and Grief: Personal Stories of Doctors and Other Healthcare Professionals*, reflected the lives being lived by the authors. Superimposed on retrieving and sharing life-changing losses was the COVID pandemic. The need for physical distancing and isolation from loved ones and the fear of violence from instigated social and racial conflict placed even greater physical, psychological, and spiritual demands on the authors. It should be noted that almost all the narrators are experts in working with seriously ill and dying patients, with many having more than thirty years of experience. Yet these were not easy stories to write, let alone share. We learned that the most valuable stories were those that were hardest to tell.

There were other invited authors who, for a variety of sound reasons, did not participate. For some, the pain remains too great to share at this time. We identified adaptive and complex evolutionary, psychological, and social inclinations which guard against exposing vulnerabilities. The authors showed great courage and resilience in breaking through these barriers, revealing the most deeply personal and intimate stories, some for the very first time, often leaving both narrator and reader with unresolved feelings. The stories recounted were memories of emotionally rich experiences: loss continues to be molded and revised in the memory as time and feelings help defend against the overwhelming pain. The act of conscious/unconscious retrieval, conjuring our ever-evolving memories of what objectively happened, becomes even more precarious and, with this continuous reprocessing, even more fascinating. Some of us had overstuffed closets of memory-stories that, once acknowledged, threatened to tumble out uncontrollably. For others, the memories had more of an impatient assertive presence, sitting vigilantly on shoulders, ready to erupt with even the slightest shift of courageous attention and opportunity.

How does one write about loss, a universal yet unique experience, without escaping into platitudes, magical thinking, or scholarly intellectualizations that loss is merely the spark that ignites grief? *Loss and Grief: Personal Stories of Doctors and Other Healthcare Professionals,* both as adventure and ordeal, had its genesis in the fact that, historically, almost all that is published, even when loss is in the title, does not define—never mind address—loss as a lingering experience. The paucity of academic exploration of loss particularly amplifies the conflation of the two distinct but related concepts of loss and grief. Significant loss is itself immutable, but, unlike the emotional aspects of grief, its meaning and power may not dissipate over time. It is a given that grief is a *response* to loss. But what is *loss*?

Loss comes to us in many forms and throughout the life cycle, such as body parts lost by accident or intention during surgery[1] or the slower, natural, inevitable losses inherent to aging that can be just as difficult to accommodate. Loss of a loved person, held with or without ambivalence, triggers inchoate emotions and reactions beyond what we have ever conceived of in ourselves. Whatever the source, loss, inevitably and forever, can alter the expected trajectory of all the lives significantly touched by the experience. The denial of its power can lead to significantly stilted emotional growth, often traumatizing in clear or unsuspected ways.

Although loss is complex and may be the most distressing of emotionally charged experiences, it is not a phantasm. Consciousness may be altered, but it is not absent. Loss is a fully biopsychosocial and, for many people, spiritual response, engendering one of the most challenging human experiences. There can be no question that the death of a loved one causes significant and simultaneous biopsychosocial disruptions. At the same time, none of these systems shuts down completely. Central and peripheral nervous systems continue to function despite the influx of confusing and overwhelming cognitive and emotional stimulation. People vary widely in how they interpret the loss as it is happening. There is consciousness during the entire loss

---

[1] Viorst, J. (2010). *Necessary losses: The loves illusions dependencies and impossible expectations that all of us must give up to grow.* New York: Simon and Schuster.

experience. There are continued body functions. There is language. There are early attempts at making meaning, making sense of the insensible. How a person might cope depends on their prior experiences with loss(s) at different developmental stages, cognitive and emotional capacities, personality traits, defenses of the self, and their psychological and social supports. Some universal questions in various forms, such as those listed below, are an attempt to regain a sense of personal control. The questions do not necessarily occur in any orderly, coherent fashion, sometimes appearing at the most inconvenient moments. Responses may differ depending on personality, developmental age, psychological mindedness, and spiritual orientation.

- What is happening?
- How can this be happening?
- Can I stop it?
- Who do I call?
- Where is the deceased now?
- Do they feel anything?
- How can the world go on when mine is disintegrating?

To our knowledge, there is no universally accepted academic definition of serious loss. Parkes and Markus, in their classic 1998 textbook, *Coping with loss: Helping patients and their families*, remark, "Why should it be that a topic that is so central in importance receives so little attention today? . . . One answer may be the assumption that the loss is irreversible and untreatable; there is nothing we can do about it, and the best way of dealing with it is to ignore it."[2] Of note is the absence, in this classic and most other textbooks, of a working definition of loss. In some ways, loss as an event is omnipresent but is also strewn across the academic landscape with no home. Parkes and Markus present a formulation which we must question: "Although the moment of death is usually a time of great distress, this is usually quickly repressed and, in Western Society, the impact is soon followed by a period of numbness which lasts for hours or days." As the stories you have just read demonstrate, loss is more than a momentary yield sign on the way to grief. Loss is the story; grief, the response.

---

[2] Parkes, C. M., & Markus, A. (1998). *Coping with loss: Helping patients and their families* (p. 3). London: BMJ.

We therefore promulgate the following definition of loss:

It is the realization of a permanent, uncontrollable, irrevocable, and undesirable separation from highly valued relationships resulting in changes in one's identity and sense of place in the universe. The primary loss almost always sets into motion a further cascade of social as well as emotional consequences.

Reduced financial resources, greater caregiving duties, smaller supportive social networks, and diminution in social status are some of the most common consequences.

Opportunities for Research and Education

Loss is more—or has the potential to be more—than the reflex that triggers grief. Despite the inevitable losses that people endure at every stage of the life cycle, most of the literature and powerful rituals are focused on grief. We ask: Where are the social, physical, psychological, or spiritual preparations for *anticipating and managing loss*? The study of grief is extremely important and there are superb textbooks and articles that have and are making major contributions to the field.[3] But we return to the question: Is the loss experience and its implications so powerfully aversive that we have abandoned any hope to be more curious about potential therapeutic advantages?

The authors' stories led to some well-trodden material that was expected, but revealed other themes that were unanticipated, if not startling. We summarize some of these themes here.

1. Having even extensive, professional expertise in helping patients and families cope with loss and grief was not at all particularly helpful in managing our own personal losses.
2. Despite the universality and inevitability of loss throughout the life cycle, there is almost no formal preparation to manage or even a language to address these realities in real time.
3. Loss almost always caused changes to one's sense of core identity and sense of place in the universe.
4. The loss experience, in retrospect, although generating sadness, longing, and pain, was also an emotional connection that few would be willing to sacrifice.

---

[3] Parkes, C. M., & Prigerson, H. G. (2013). *Bereavement: Studies of grief in adult life*. New York: Routledge.

5. There is an urgent need to normalize, anticipate, and promote healing and growth from loss and grief experiences.
6. Although the emotional response to grief almost always subsides over time, loss as a connection to the object never truly goes away.
7. Because supportive agencies, including healthcare environments, lack the infrastructure and policies to address universal, inevitable losses, they may ignore, deny, and punish when we need them most.

Loss in the Context of Healthcare Systems and Social Settings

It is no secret that it is not within the culture of medicine to openly share losses or for institutions to create the infrastructure for such support systems.[4] Paradoxically, it is not uncommon that, in some of the most supportive health systems, the very professionals who care so compassionately for patients feel so alone when they experience their own personal losses. The authors' powerful narratives and many decades in healthcare lead us to believe that supportive and palliative care programs are no different when it comes to open communication and support for colleagues experiencing life-altering losses. In fact, one of the most consistent themes early in the group processing of the evolving stories was that when the loss hit home, it did not help much, if at all, to be a highly skilled professional. This professional self, even for those who have counseled dying patients and their caregivers over many decades, felt the loss of language *when they were in it*. The surfacing of this humbling insight was highly instructive, supportive, freeing, and inspiring to the authors in being able to discuss this level of courageous vulnerability. Professional training or identity offered no immunity or direction for a loss that was deeply personal. The professional veneer was too thin to be instructive or protective. This was a surprise. Perhaps it should not have been.

Serious loss brought each of us back to the exposed core of our most basic selves. But which self? Which me are we talking about? Professional? Parent? Child? Artist? Savior? Explorer? Competitor? Victim? We are all comprised of layers of highly context-sensitive, multi-selves, sub-selves, other-selves,

[4] Harrison, K. L. (2021). Making space for grief in academia. *Journal of the American Medical Association* 326(8), 699–700.

and/or sub-personalities.[5] The roles we play and the demands of the immediate social situation have a major impact on our responses, as they do in everyday life, but only much more so when the stakes are so high. This shape-shifter potential can be a strength used, with attention and intention, to consciously enhance personal agency in deciding which parts of ourselves we want to activate, rather than inflexibly being limited to history or habit. Knowing that we have options in how to respond—*reflect over reflex*—can be an ego strength with implications for coping with loss. The behavioral and cognitive manifestations of these choices are replete throughout the stories shared.

The stories identified the dangers and stark reality of formidable barriers to addressing loss and grief in ourselves and colleagues. In fact, obstacles are even greater for the professionals who are socialized and rewarded for being "Supermen," devoid of emotions or limitations. For women, they were expected to simply act like and adapt to the privileged male model (which for them seldom existed) or abandon hopes for advancement. This gender inequality still exists.[6] Nietzsche's oft quoted trope in medicine, "*What doesn't kill me makes me stronger,*" is at best outdated, simplistic, destructive, and flies in the face of what it means to be open to the full range of human experiences.[7] Although most people do recover from even the most tragic of losses, there are some losses that inhabit such deep places in our emotional core and are so foreign to our sense of identity that full recovery is not realistic or possible. For example, the deaths of young children and sudden violent deaths are notably excruciating.[8,9]

More recently, and long overdue, increased attention is being given to the impact of social supports on loss. Losses always occur within a social milieu. An emerging literature reinforces that social and cultural aspects of loss ("social spaces") are relevant to making loss less

[5] Kenrick, D. T. (2011). *Sex, murder, and the meaning of life: A psychologist investigates how evolution, cognition, and complexity are revolutionizing our view of human nature.* New York: Basic Books.

[6] Ruzycki, S. M., Brown, A., Bharwani, A., & Freeman, G. (2021). Gender-based disparities in medicine: A theoretical framework for understanding opposition to equity and equality. *BMJ Leader*, leader-2020.

[7] Nietzsche, F. (1998). *Twilight of the idols.* Oxford: Oxford University Press.

[8] Bonanno, G. A. (2005). Resilience in the face of potential trauma. *Current Directions in Psychological Science 14*(3), 135–138. doi:10.1111/j.0963-7214.2005.00347.x.

[9] Parkes, C. M., & Prigerson, H. G. (2013). *Bereavement: Studies of grief in adult life.* New York: Routledge.

traumatic.[10,11] The impact of responses and the influence of the social milieu in which they occurred were of significant influence in almost all the narratives. Not a single narrator felt that their professional environment was prepared to prospectively provide adequate support. Although once shared with others loss and grief can engender compassionate social responses, there were also other complex emotions that arose from the writing. For example, loss and the resulting grief have long been known to create a sense of shame and fear that others may exploit the situation. "Blood in the water" ("colleagues" choosing opportunity over duty and loyalty) was a reality that surfaced early in the writing process relating to the reflections of the narrators and their past losses as well as to publishing these stories for all to see.

Still, connecting to others with shared experience is a proven, essential part of adapting to new realities caused by loss. But this can only happen if there is space for the loss to be known. Too often, as we learned, this is not the case. Doctors and other healthcare professionals are deeply committed to helping and healing others. In the emotionally charged context of unremitting loss, too much is expected: demanding and unrealistic work schedules (too little time to see too many patients), managing the complex emotional reactions of patients and families, striving to see patients within their unique personal and social situations, being confronted with problems that cannot be solved only mitigated, deciphering intricate interactions with colleagues who have higher and lower status, and, finally, attempting to have some semblance of a personal and family life.

We ask, as have many others: Where is the humanity in medicine? How did we ever get to a place where a colleague needing time off to care for two special needs children is a "special case"? This putative "special case" is neither unusual nor special. It is not possible to make clear distinctions between personal and professional life; this is a nonfunctional myth, compounded by inherent gender inequality. Women sleep less and do more than men as it relates to family. Most professionals in healthcare are women, and that number continues to increase. How is it that we do not have systematic ways and existing institutional infrastructure to support women and men when

[10] Maciejewski, P. K., Falzarano, F. B., She, W. J., Lichtenthal, W. G., & Prigerson, H. G. (July 7, 2021). A micro-sociological theory of adjustment to loss. *Current Opinions in Psychology 43*, 96–101. doi: 10.1016/j.copsyc.2021.06.016. Epub ahead of print. PMID: 34333375.

[11] Prigerson, H. G., Kakarala, S., Gang, J., & Maciejewski, P. K. (2021). History and status of prolonged grief disorder as a psychiatric diagnosis. *Annual Review of Clinical Psychology, 17*, 109–126.

they experience such expected challenges—never mind, traumatizing personal losses?

Summary and a Way Forward

As revealed in the heroic stories within and superimposed on the prolonged COVID pandemic-created zeitgeist, we are a long way from making healthcare healthier, more realistic to the needs of the actual workforce, and compassionate. In some ways, we may be going in the wrong direction. The psychological barriers for individuals who cannot share their own losses and distress with colleagues reflects a society that denies the impact of loss and minimizes the emotional components of vulnerabilities. It does not have to be this way.

Thinking forward, can we create developmentally age-appropriate and culturally tailored language to detoxify the most isolating aspects of loss? Can we create a language for the loss experience that is strengths-based and healing? Are there ways to normalize inevitable loss and suffering? How can we objectively question and explore the prevailing assumption that the loss experience is simply a triggering event for the grief response? Does being actively in the eye of the hurricane of loss really preclude seeing a wider perspective and options? Perhaps our most immediate goal could be to create an infrastructure within healthcare to best support healthcare professionals in managing the relentless professional stream of losses and personal suffering.

It is ironic that at a time when there is so much talk about moral injury and distress there is less time to do anything about it. A healthier more supportive workforce is an investment, not a cost. What are the personal and societal implications for how people will live (with attention/intention) when they have access to age-appropriate and culturally sensitive ongoing conversations about loss? How can we not better prepare people for something that is inevitable, universal, and life-altering? How can anything so important as loss and grief be left to chance and not taught formally? By acknowledging that we will inevitably lose all that we value most—family, partners, status, our own lives—can we open doors for greater personal and social maturity? Is there something to be learned from the anticipated sadness and suffering? Is it realistic to expect that pre-learning in a language that is age-appropriate and culturally tailored about loss events can become a bridge to internal and social support systems that enhance mental, physical, and spiritual health?

We are aware that we are asking for perhaps the impossible: to make and keep conscious in all of us the ever-present fragility of life to prepare us for the universal experience of loss. Biological and psychological evolution has left us with powerful defenses of denial as well as those that allow us to live and grow in the face of the ultimate loss of those loved and of ourselves. It is our hope that reading these deeply personal stories and such openly shared feelings of isolation and suffering will not only humanize the loss experience, but ignite prospective discussions and illuminate opportunities for education, research, and resulting interventions to prepare us for the multiple small and large loss experiences endemic to life.

Doctors and other healthcare professionals must face pain in their own lives, disrupting the fantasy that somehow they are immune to loss and grief while they care for others. Sometimes that disruption is so profound that it destroys careers and relationships. This book has been a work of great sacrifice as each author worked through their own loss and grief in the writing of their narrative. We are so grateful for their courage and willingness to bare their pain and suffering as they bear the profound changes in each heart, soul, and life.

The unflinching, deeply personal stories of loss and grief shared by the narrators, who had the audacity to *walk their own shoes*, are as powerful as they are sad. These are universal memory stories from the frontline of life about how we perceive, make sense of, and grow with core losses. There are many questions yet to be addressed, but, ultimately, we must ask: If doctors and other healthcare professionals are not at the vanguard of making a world filled with loss and grief more loving and kind, who will be?

Suggested Reading

American Association of Hospice and Palliative Medicine. (2022). Statement on diversity, equity & inclusion. https://aahpm.org/membership/diversity.

Back, A. L., Young, J. P., McCown, E., Engelberg, R. A., Vig, E. K., Reinke, L. F., Wenrich, M. D., McGrath, B. B., & Curtis, J. R. (March 9, 2009). Abandonment at the end of life from patient, caregiver, nurse and physician perspectives: Loss of continuity and lack of closure. *Archives of Internal Medicine 9*, 169(5), 474–479. doi:10.1001/archinternmed.2008.583.

Balboni, T., & Balboni, M. (2019). From hostility to hospitality. In Anthony L. Back, Jessica P. Young, Ellen McCown, Ruth A. Engelberg, Elizabeth K. Vig, Lynn F. Reinke, Marjorie D. Wenrich, Barbara B. McGrath, and J. Randall Curtis (Eds.), *Hostility to hospitality: Spirituality and professional socialization within medicine* (pp. 296–314). New York: Oxford University Press.

Berger, A. M., & O'Neill, J. F. (2021). *Principles and practice of palliative care and supportive oncology* (5th ed.). Philadelphia: Lippincott.

Bitz, C., Kent, E. E., Clark, K., & Loscalzo, M. (2020). Couples coping with cancer together: Successful implementation of a caregiver program as standard of care. *Psycho-Oncology 29*, 902–909. https://doi.org/10.1002/pon.5364.

Bonanno, G. A. (2005). Resilience in the face of potential trauma. *Current Directions in Psychological Science 14*(3), 135–138. doi:10.1111/j.0963-7214.2005.00347.x.

Bonanno, G. A. (2019). *The other side of sadness: What the new science of bereavement tells us about life after loss.* Paris: Hachette.

Bonanno, G. A. (2021). *The end of trauma: How the new science of resilience is changing how we think about PTSD.* Paris: Hachette.

Bucher, J., Houts, P., & Ades, T. (2011). *American Cancer Society complete guide to family caregiving: The essential guide to cancer caregiving at home.* Atlanta, GA: American Cancer Society/Health Promotions.

Cassel, E. (2013). "What Is Healing?" and "Listening." In Eric Cassell (Ed.), *The nature of healing: The modern practice of medicine* (pp. 81–114). New York: Oxford University Press.

Dysvik, E., & Furnes, B. (2010). Dealing with grief related to loss by death and chronic pain: Suggestions for practice. Part 2. *Patient Preference and Adherence 4*, 163–170. doi:10.2147/ppa.s10582.

Emanuel, L., & Librach, S. (2007). *Palliative care: Core skills and clinical competencies.* Philadelphia, PA: Saunders/Elsevier.

Emanuel, L., & Librach, S. (2011). *Palliative care: Core skills and clinical competencies.* Philadelphia, PA: Saunders.

Field, M. J., & Cassel, C. K. (Eds.). (1997). *Approaching death: Improving care at the end of life.* Washington, DC: Institute of Medicine/National Academy of Sciences.

Folkman, S. (2011). *The Oxford handbook of stress, health, and coping.* New York: Oxford University Press.

Frankl, V. (2006). *Man's search for meaning.* New York: Beacon Press.

Gawande, A. (2014). *Being mortal.* New York: Metropolitan Books.

Grassi, L., & Riba, M. (2012). *Clinical psycho-oncology: An international perspective.* London: Wiley.

Hart, O. (1983). *Rituals in psychotherapy: Transition and continuity.* North Stratford, NH: Irvington Publishers.

Hitchens, C., Carter, G., & Blue, C. (2014). *Mortality.* New York: Twelve.

Holmes, J. (1993). *John Bowlby and attachment theory.* London: Routledge.

Irwin, K. E., & Loscalzo, M. L. (2020). Witnessing unnecessary suffering: A call for action and policy change to increase access to psycho-oncology care. *Psycho-oncology 29*(12), 1977–1981. https://doi.org/10.1002/pon.5599.

Kim, P. Y., & Loscalzo, M. J. (Eds.). (2018). *Gender in psycho-oncology.* New York: Oxford University Press.

Kleinman, A. (1988). *The illness narratives.* New York: Basic Books.

Lamas, D. J. (2020). Families are central to critical care: But the waiting room is empty. New York Times (Opinion Guest Essay). https://www.nytimes.com/2020/08/17/opinion/coronavirus-hopsitals-visitors.html.

Lamas, D. J. (2020). My patients will not be the same: None of us will. New York Times (Opinion Guest Essay). https://www.nytimes.com/2021/05/19/opinion/pandemic-mental-health.html.

Lamas, D. J. (2020). To my patients' family members. New York Times (Doctors). https://www.nytimes.com/2020/05/20/well/live/coronavirus-patients-families-hospital-visits-doctors-apology.html.

Leiter, R. (2020). Reentry. *New England Journal of Medicine* 383:e141 doi:10.1056/NEJMp2027447.

Lidz, T. (1983). *The person, his and her development throughout the life cycle.* New York: Basic Books.

Loscalzo, M., & Clark, K. (2018). Gender opportunities in psychosocial oncology. In Matthew Clark & Karen Clark (Eds.), *Psycho-oncology* (pp. 35–55). Cham, SW: Springer.

Loscalzo, M., Clark, K., Bitz, C., Rosenstein, D., & Yopp, J. (2018). When the invisible screen becomes visible: Sex and gender matters in biopsychosocial interventions and programs. In Y. Kim & M. Loscalzo (Eds.), *Gender-oriented psycho-oncology: Research and practice* (pp. 35–55). New York: Oxford University Press.

Loscalzo, M. J., Kim, Y., & Clark, K. C. (2010). Gender and caregiving. In J. Holland et al. (Eds.), *Textbook of psycho-oncology* (2nd ed.; pp. 522–526). New York: Oxford University Press.

Loscalzo, M. J., & Von Gunten, C. (2009). Interdisciplinary teamwork in palliative care: Compassionate expertise for serious illness. In H. M. Chochinov & W. Breitbart (Eds.), *Handbook of psychiatry in palliative medicine* (2nd ed.; pp. 172–185). New York: Oxford University Press.

Maciejewski, P. K., Falzarano, F. B., She, W. J., Lichtenthal, W. G., & Prigerson, H. G. (2021 July 7). A micro-sociological theory of adjustment to loss. *Current Opinions in Psychology 43*, 96–101. doi:10.1016/j.copsyc.2021.06.016. Epub ahead of print. PMID: 34333375.

Maguire, P., & Parkes, C. M. (1998). Coping with loss: Surgery and loss of body parts. *British Medical Journal 316*(7137), 1086.

Montross-Thomas, L. P., Scheiber, C., Meier, E. A., & Irwin, S. A. (2016). Personally mean-ingful rituals: A way to increase compassion and decrease burnout among hospice staff and volunteers. *Journal of Palliative Medicine 19*, 10.

O'Connor, M. F. (2022). *The grieving brain: The surprising science of how we learn from love and loss*. New York: Harper One.

Papa, A., Lancaster, N. G., & Kahler, J. (2014 June 14). Commonalities in grief responding across bereavement and non-bereavement losses. *Journal of Affective Disorders 161*, 136–143. doi:10.1016/j.jad.2014.03.018. Epub Mar 25, 2014.

Parkes, C. M. (1998). Bereavement in adult life. *British Medical Journal 316*(7134), 856–859.

Parkes, C. M., & Markus, A. (1998). *Coping with loss: Helping patients and their families*. London: BMJ.

Parkes, C. M., & Prigerson, H. G. (2013). *Bereavement: Studies of grief in adult life*. New York: Routledge.

Prigerson, H. G., Kakarala, S., Gang, J., & Maciejewski, P. K. (2021). History and status of prolonged grief disorder as a psychiatric diagnosis. *Annual Review of Clinical Psychology 17*, 109–126.

Richo, D. (2005). *The five things we cannot change: And the happiness we find by embracing them*. Boston, MA: Shambhala.

Rosenstein, D. L., & Yopp, J. M. (2018). *The group: Seven widowed fathers reimagine life*. New York: Oxford University Press.

Stroebe, M., & Schut, H. (2010). The dual process model of coping with bereavement: A decade on. *OMEGA Journal of Death and Dying 61*(4), 273–289.

Stroebe, M., & Schut, H. (2021). Bereavement in times of COVID-19: A review and theo-retical framework. *OMEGA Journal of Death and Dying 82*(3), 500–522.

Thompson, N. (2002). *Loss and grief: A guide for human services practitioners*. Houndsmills, UK: Palgrave.

Viorst, J. (1986). *Necessary losses*. New York: Simon and Schuster.

Walter, C., & McCoyd, J. (2016). *Grief and loss across the lifespan: A biopsychosocial per-spective*. New York: Springer.

White-Davis, T., Edgoose, J., Brown Speights, J. S., Fraser, K., Ring, J. M., Guh, J., & Saba, G. W. (2018 May). Addressing racism in medical education: An interactive training module. *Family Medicine 50*(5), 364–368. doi:10.22454/FamMed.2018.875510. PMID: 29762795.

Young, K. (Ed.). (2013). *The art of losing: Poems of grief and healing*. New York: Bloomsbury USA.

Zabora, J., & Loscalzo, M. (2021). Psychosocial consequences of advanced cancer. In A. Berger & J. F. O'Neill (Eds.), *Principles and practice of palliative care and support on-cology* (pp. 626–644). Philadelphia: Lippincott.

Index